GET HEALTHY NOW FOR LIFE

GET HEALTHY NOW FOR LIFE

Published in the United States by:
Ryan and Monica Wohlfert, P.C.
Total Health Chiropractic
252 S. Waverly Road
Lansing, MI 48917

Photos by Shirley Wohlfert

DISCLAIMER

The information contained in this book is based upon the research and personal and professional experiences of the author. It is not intended as a substitute for consulting with your physician or other health care providers. Any attempt to diagnose and treat an illness should be done under the direction of a health care professional. The author and publisher do not advocate the use of any particular health care protocol but believe this information should be available to the public. The author and publisher are also not responsible in any manner whatsoever for any injury, adverse effects, or consequences that may occur through following the instructions in this material. The activities described in this book are for informational purposes and may be too strenuous for some people. Please consult your physician if they are too strenuous or dangerous for the reader to perform. If you cannot agree to the above, please do not read this book.

GET HEALTHY
NOW
FOR LIFE

RYAN WOHLFERT, DC, CSCS, CCSP

This book is dedicated to my girls – my wife Monica and our three awesome little girls, Rylee, Dylan, and Kaelyn. They motivate me to be a lifelong learner so I can be a lifelong teacher.

ACKNOWLEDGEMENTS

I want to thank everyone who has taught me about health, wellness, and life.

First and foremost is my family: my wife Monica; little girls Rylee, Dylan, and Kaelyn; my mom and dad, Toni and Stan; and my brothers, Tyler, Adam, and Jordan.

My wife and I have the greatest T.E.A.M. at Total Health Chiropractic and it would be a huge mistake if I didn't thank them for making our days run as smoothly and successfully as they do: Lori Briedenstein, Erica Green, Annette Humphries, Cara Nemeth, Amy Wirth, Dr. Sara Young, and Dr. Tom Sandberg. With your help, we accomplish our goal of making a positive difference in every life we touch.

I've had many great teachers over the years like Ron Kramer, Brian Grasso, Mike Boyle, Dr. Rodger Massa, Dr. Jim Jedlicka, Dr. John Wycoff, Lee Taft, Dr. Evan Osar, and Gray Cook.

I want to make special mention of three lifelong friends: Ted Arens, Joe Keilen, and Dan Kushner. I know that no matter what happens, we will always be there for each other.

"Work harder on yourself than you do on your job." I want to thank the following great individuals for teaching me that principle and "to get everything you want, help as many people as possible get what they want." Jim Rohn, Zig Ziglar, Chris Widener, John Maxwell, Ryan Lee, Dr. Wayne Dyer, Russell Brunson, and John Wooden are a few names that come to mind.

This is just the start of something bigger.

Yours in Health,

Ryan L Wohlfert, DC, CSCS, CCSP

CONTENTS

What is Health?..14

Achieve Physical Balance and Alignment............................28

Exercise: Life is Movement..42

Nutrition Basics:
Pro-Inflammation vs. Anti-inflammation.............................96

Mental Balance and Alignment:
De-stress, not Distress...113

Children's Health:
What They Aren't Telling You..128

Stressor List..152

Frequently Asked Questions..161

Total Health Recommends...182

INTRODUCTION

I don't have a big dramatic story, and I don't have a life-changing experience. The truth is, I've always been healthy and active. I've had injuries in the past, but nothing that's limited my activities. Many books and fitness programs out there are from people who have hit rock bottom and had to change their lives to survive. Maybe they have been hooked on drugs, or have been 100 pounds overweight. But that's not me. I have had ups and downs, bumps, and bruises along the way, but have never allowed myself to hit rock bottom. And I don't plan to. I empathize with those who experience dramatic health issues. You can definitely learn from others who have brought themselves back up, but wouldn't it be smart to listen to someone who knows how to keep from getting to that point? Absolutely! Let's say you are unhealthy and are sliding down that slope. The principles and action steps in *Get Healthy Now for Life* still apply to you. This is a practical, easy to understand guide to health.

America's health is not good. In 2007, we spent $2.2 trillion on healthcare, which is an average of $7,421 per person, per year. The secret is, you can prevent many of the health problems that are bankrupting America today: Heart disease, cancer, diabetes, depression, chronic pain, and obesity. These are called chronic preventable diseases. But you have to put the work in to prevent or rid yourself of chronic illness. If you don't want to put in the work, don't read this book. It's not that it's hard to do, but it's a change. It's different than what you're used to, but if you're willing to give six little, measly months to your health, this guide is for you.

Just because something has been done a certain way for years, doesn't mean it's the right way to do it today. If that were the case, we would still be using typewriters. We would still be wearing Chuck Taylor basketball shoes. We would still be using the old golf clubs. As bestselling author Harvey McKay states a, "good leader understands that anything that has been done in a particular way for a given amount of time is being done wrong." In America's health care, things have been done a certain way for a period of time, but that does not mean it is giving us healthy results. Dr. Barbara Starfield, from Johns Hopkins Bloomberg School of Public Health, conducted a study about why our health is so poor. One finding was the U.S. population accounts for five percent of the world's population, yet we consume 60% of the prescription medications in the world. This was her conclusion: "Prescription drugs and medical treatments have not only failed to improve the health of Americans, but have also led to the decline in the overall well-being of Americans."

Dr. Starfield, a distinguished professor and medical doctor, is saying this about the medical profession. Her findings even appeared in *The Journal of the American Medical Association*, so why aren't things changing in the health care system? Drugs and medical treatment have their place, but it seems they have lost their way.

My purpose, career, and this book, are based on something very simple, but not easy: *If you improve your health, many (or all) of your symptoms and diseases will go away.* Here is some proof. If you have ever watched *The Biggest Loser* television show, you understand that point. There are overweight and obese people who go to a ranch and learn to exercise, eat nutritious foods, improve their self-image, and balance their bodies. Before they start, they get a physical and give the doctor all the medications they are taking for high blood pressure, diabetes, depression, high cholesterol, chronic pain, asthma, and on and on. Then they begin doing healthy activities, lose some weight, and get healthier. During this process, their blood pressure and cholesterol move into the normal range without medication; their diabetes and depression are under control with minimal or no medication; their pain and asthma are gone! All of these conditions are classified as diseases, but the doctor says something very logical (at least to me). When they lost weight and got healthier, he said, "All these drugs were doing was covering up the cause of these diseases…which is your poor health." Bingo! Everyone wants someone else to pay for their health, but the truth is you have to put in the time, and sometimes the money, to get healthy. It's up to you; no one else.

Prescription drugs and medical treatments are not the only reason America's health is deteriorating. *Get Healthy Now for Life* examines the myriad reasons and the action steps you can take to improve your health, and America's health. It is up to you, no one else, to put in the time (and sometimes the money) to get healthy now and live the life you've always dreamed.

Yours in Health,

Ryan Wohlfert, DC, CSCS, CCSP

WHAT IS HEALTH?

HEALTH IS CONFUSING SOMETIMES. You hear it all the time, but do you really know what being healthy means? Maybe it's easier to explain what health is not. Health is not just being pain free. Similarly, an absence of poverty doesn't mean you're wealthy. You may think if you don't have pain, that you're healthy. However, think about all the things that don't cause pain or other symptoms until it's been building for years, such as high blood pressure, high cholesterol, cancer, diabetes, arthritis, obesity, and depression. You cannot rely on how you feel to determine your health.

Health is your body working at its optimum level, physically, mentally, emotionally, chemically, and even spiritually. If you take drugs or medication, you are not healthy. Drugs do not make you healthy. They just treat the symptoms. Drugs just cover up the **cause** of the symptoms, which is usually poor health. For example, if you've ever watched the show, *The Biggest Loser*, the contestants start off on the ranch overweight and unhealthy. They receive their standard physical exam, and a review of all the medications they are taking for their different ailments like high blood pressure, high cholesterol, asthma, diabetes, or reflux. When they lose as little as 10 to 15% of their body weight, many of those symptoms go away and they do not have to take their medication anymore. The doctor actually says, "All these drugs are doing is covering up the real cause of those problems, and that is poor health."

The best definition of health I can come up with was adapted from Jim Rohn's quote about success and failure: "All health is, is a few disciplines practiced every day, while disease and symptoms are a few errors in judgment repeated every day. Whether you are healthy or have disease, it is essentially the accumulation of daily disciplines and errors in judgment."

Why is America's Health so Bad?

You need to understand what **causes** the symptoms and disease in the first place. Three factors cause your body to develop these symptoms: Physical stress, chemical stress, and emotional and mental stress that we put on our body.

Physical Stress

Physical stress you put on your body could include past accidents, falls, injuries, serious medical ailments, sports injuries, performing repetitive movements, improper bending techniques, or sitting down at a computer for long periods of time. In addition, _not_ exercising, stretching, getting massages, receiving chiropractic adjustments, or getting adequate sleep increases your body's physical stress. Many Americans have white-collar jobs where they sit all day. That is a great physical stress to explain. Your body was designed to move. When you are sedentary, your posture gets poor, muscles get tight, and nerves get irritated, which puts more stress on your body and causes it to break down.

Chemical Stress

Chemical stress is any unhealthy food, drink, or drug you put into your body, as well as any nutritious food or drink that you omit. For example, processed food, fast food, caffeine, nicotine, alcohol, sugar, drugs, and medications are all chemical stresses that you put into your body. Failing to eat raw fruits and vegetables, drink water, eat breakfast, or take vitamins also constitutes a chemical stress.

Dr. Barbara Starfield, MD had interesting conclusions in the *Journal the of the American Medical Association* in 2000. First, she determined the United State's population accounts for 5% of the world's population, but we consume 60% of the prescription medications in the world! She concluded, "prescription drugs, medical treatments, have not only failed to improve the health of Americans, but also led to the decline in the overall well-being of Americans."

Drugs are a chemical stress. Does that mean you should throw away your medication? No! Find out why you are taking these medications in the first place. Recall *The Biggest Loser* example. They may be taking these medications for the same conditions as you, and just like you, those medications are just covering up the symptoms of poor health. Once you address the root cause and get healthy, many (or all) symptoms and diseases vanish.

Emotional & Mental Stress

Emotional or mental stress is what most of us think about when we say, "I am so stressed!" Your mental stress could include financial problems, work issues, challenges in getting along with people, family, being happy with yourself, or your future. Other sources of mental stress are being cynical and disenchanted, irritable and short tempered, mentally sluggish, or having poor concentration. This stress may be the most severe because many times it is insidious. You do not know what is happening because you have not done anything physically different. But over time, mental stress exhibits itself as physical symptoms such as headaches, a stiff neck, tight shoulders and back muscles, stomachaches, or ulcers. To treat these physical symptoms, you have to manage the mental stresses.

Americans in general experience enormous amounts of physical, chemical, and emotional (mental) stresses. Could that be why America's health is so poor? Absolutely! These stresses cause your body to get out of balance. For example, with physical imbalances (such as poor posture or structure), more stress is on your nerves, muscles, joints, and bones, which makes your body work harder. Over time, this repeated stress leads to the breakdown of those structures, and then causes symptoms and disease. If you are just treating the symptoms, and not removing the cause, then you will continue to have poor health.

You may be asking yourself, "What about genetics? Isn't that the cause?" Without going into detail about the science of genetics, which is beyond the scope of this book, your genes will not determine whether you have heart disease, cancer, obesity, or arthritis. Through the research of Dr. Lipton and other leading-edge scientists, new discoveries have been made about the interaction between your mind and body and the processes by which cells receive information. It shows that genes and DNA **do not** control our biology, that instead DNA is controlled by signals from outside the cell, i.e. physical, chemical, and emotional stresses. This is called the study of *epi*genetics. This is reassuring news since we can manage our environment and what we do, eat, and think. Therefore, we are not at the mercy of our genetics and can control our own health!

How Do We Fix It?

Now that you know the problem that causes poor health and disease, the question arises, how do we fix it? It is up to you to improve this problem. It is up to you to improve your health. We all talk about how health is the most important thing in our lives, but we don't spend a lot of our time or money on our health. Yes, we just spent $2.2 trillion, but that's not spent on getting and staying healthy. That is spent on the consequences of us not being healthy; the diagnosis and treatment of the diseases caused by poor health like heart disease, cancer, chronic pain, diabetes, and obesity.

Your Beliefs

The first step to getting healthy is determining your beliefs about health. Is it too hard to perform healthy activities? Is it no fun? Do you not have time? Do you know *why* you have those beliefs? Do you know *how* to get healthy? Do you know *what* to do?

Secondly, do you believe you can be healthy? Some people believe that because of genetics they cannot do it. "My mom has high blood pressure so I'm going to have high blood pressure." Maybe you are not receiving, or feel you will not receive, support from your family and friends. Television and the media show images that you feel are unattainable. Take your foot off the brake to your health! You can learn all of the how-to's, but unless you know why you do not engage in healthy activities, you will not change your beliefs. You can deal with all of these obstacles and get healthy by changing your beliefs about the activities necessary to get healthy.

Change Your Beliefs, Change Your Behavior

Once you identify your beliefs and change them, you will change your behavior. If you try to change your behavior first, you greatly increase your chance of a relapse. Your beliefs are the "why" and your behaviors are the "how."

A big problem is equating healthy activities with pain. You *have* to do things that you do not like to do. Unfortunately, many people anchor pleasure to unhealthy things that are fleeting, like eating cake, ice cream, chocolate, watching television, smoking, and not exercising. Those things make you feel good for a little while, but then you beat yourself up about them later. Therefore, you need to reverse those beliefs. Anchor some pleasure to healthy activities and pain to unhealthy things.

Perform a cost versus benefits analysis of what you do to your body. What stresses do you put on your body that will cause it to get diseased? Physiologically, what are they doing to your organs, bones, muscles, and brain? How are you going to feel afterwards, if you do that particular activity? How are you going to feel the next day? Answering those questions will anchor pain to the activity. For the benefits or pleasure, how would your body feel if you refrained from performing some of your unhealthy activities for the next month, two months, or even six months?

Address how exercising moderately, eating nutritious food, thinking healthy, and having physical balance will make you feel. Ask yourself, "What part of my life would stink if I had to give up something bad for me; the five minutes where I had to give it up, or the other 23 hours and 55 minutes of the day?" Link pleasure to the good and pain to the bad, and that will change your behavior. Noted self-improvement guru

20

Brian Tracy accurately states the need to "resolve to be a master of change rather than a victim of change."

Assess Your Readiness to Change

It is a Catch-22. You need to do some work to get healthy, but you got unhealthy because you did not do the work. Therefore, you must make changes. You must want to change. This will assess your readiness to change.

Prochaska and DiClemente's Stages of Change model was developed after alcoholism killed James Prochaska's father. Prochaska resolved to find a way to help people break their bad habits. Prochaska, a renowned psychologist at the University of Rhode Island and author of *Changing for Good,* found ordinary people who had dropped bad habits, like smoking and overeating, on their own. After years of studying these successful changers, Prochaska detected a pattern. No matter what habit they had broken, self-changers had all progressed through the same six stages along the way. They also used a unique set of strategies at each stage.

Prochaska's approach, commonly known as the "Stages of Change" model, is simple and powerful. First, you have to find your stage, and then the model tells you what to do next. Sometimes Prochaska's self-changers would fall back a stage or two, but once they resumed the strategies specific to their stage, they would be back on track. "The only mistake you can make is to give up on yourself," Prochaska says.

21

Though Prochaska's studies focused on drug abusers, his approach is a powerful tool for people wanting to get healthy. Here is how it can help you get moving.

Stage 1: Precontemplation: "Ignorance is Bliss"

Precontemplators have not yet decided to make a change. You know exercise and eating nutritious food is healthy, but you are not quite convinced the benefits outweigh the trouble of getting started.

Action Step: Put On Your Thinking Cap

- This is not the time to "just do it." Instead, start educating yourself about how doing healthy things like exercising, eating clean, and getting physically and mentally balanced will benefit you. Start with a tip from Prochaska: "Your couch can kill you."
- List your reasons for wanting to get healthy and weigh these benefits against the consequences of staying sedentary. You need to associate "pain" with your unhealthy activities. Once your pluses outnumber the minuses, you will be ready to move forward.

I can understand why you may be in this stage and I don't want to preach to you. You are an adult and you will be the one to decide if and when you are ready to get healthy. Everyone who has ever been unhappy with their health starts right where you are now. They start by seeing the reasons why they might want to lose weight, live longer, live better, or be pain free. It is totally up to you to decide if this is best for you right now.

Stage 2: Contemplation: "Sitting on the Fence"
You're seriously considering change, but you're not ready to start yet. This is a stage of inertia and some people spend years stuck here, so relax. Your next step is planning. You might say: "Yes, my health is a concern for me, but I'm not willing or able to begin taking action within the next month." If you keep sliding back to the contemplation stage, it's probably because you jumped straight into action too soon, so DON'T jump to the action stage yet.

Action Step: Figure Out What's Blocking You
- Take an honest look at what's really preventing you from getting started. Do you think it will be too hard? Do you think you won't accomplish your goal?
- Get committed. Promise yourself you'll overcome those obstacles. Keep in mind "why" you want to get healthy. What will your life be like?

If you feel you would like to make some changes, the next step won't be jumping into action. It will begin with some preparation work.

Stage 3: Preparation: "Testing the Waters"

You realize your health is a concern for you. You are clear that the benefits of attempting healthy actions outweigh the drawbacks, and are planning to start within the next month.

You've made a commitment and you're planning to take action soon, probably within the next month.

Action Step: Make Yourself a Plan

- Think through all the details. Will you walk or swim? Where and when will you exercise? What kind of clothing or equipment do you need? What foods are healthy? Which healthy food can you most easily substitute for unhealthy food?
- Draw up a contract with yourself and set three goals. One for the next month, one for six months, and one for twelve months. For example, if weight loss is desired, a short-term goal could be, "I will lose two pounds per week for the next four weeks." Reward yourself for each goal accomplished. Set an initial goal you are sure to attain; early success will propel you onward.
- Develop a detailed contingency plan to limit excuses as much as possible. Where will you walk if it rains? How will you exercise when you visit your in-laws? What will you do on days when you are tired?
- Make a public commitment. Ask for support from your friends and have them follow up on your progress. Which family members or friends could

support you as you make this change? In what way might they support you?

Stage 4: Action: "Just Doing It"

You're taking action now and actually implementing your new fitness plan. This is where the proverbial rubber meets the road. Your preparation is put into action.

Action Steps: Put Your Plan in Motion
- Make your environment conducive to a healthy lifestyle. Leave notes reminding yourself to work out, have lists of healthy foods, keep a journal with positive affirmations, and be aware of your posture when you look in the mirror.
- Reward yourself for sticking to your plan.
- Combat feelings of loss by thinking of the long-term benefits. You are forming a lifelong habit here. No need to fret about a missed day. You have the next 50 years to make it up.

Stage 5: Maintenance: "You Know You Can Do It"

You have been making healthy lifestyle changes regularly for six months, and now you realize you can do it.

Action Steps: Work Out the Kinks
- Create a new and positive mental image of yourself. See yourself tall and strong, exercising, eating well,

and thinking healthy. Visualize this new image often. This "healthy identity" will help the habits stick.
- Learn from your mistakes, and figure out how to avoid them next time.
- Watch for the benefits and results to appear -- less huffing and puffing, more energy -- and relish them.

Stage 6: Termination: "You've Done It"

You have terminated your sedentary habits and replaced them with healthy ones. It's the end of the inactive you. You've done it!

Action Step: Pat yourself on the back
- Take a moment and acknowledge your achievement. Realize you've created new health habits that are going to serve and benefit you for life.
- Keep doing what you're doing!
- Reinforce your new habits by surrounding yourself with others with similar health habits.

Relapse: "Falling From Grace"

Some of you may experience relapse. This is the resumption of old behaviors, which is all too common. "Falling back into old habits."

Action Step: Evaluate the trigger for the relapse
- Was there something specific or did it happen gradually?
- Recall how good you felt reaching your goals, feeling great, and living healthy.

- Plan a stronger coping strategy to deal with these issues if they come up again.

Just because you fell off the horse does not mean you cannot get back on. It's likely to be much easier to get back on track because you know how. You've accomplished it before, and you can do it again! Never give up!

ACHIEVE PHYSICAL BALANCE AND ALIGNMENT

WHEN THINKING ABOUT HEALTH and fitness, physical balance may not even come to mind for most people. However, it is just as important to your health as exercise, nutrition, and healthy thinking. How does your alignment, that is posture, relate to your health? Everything breaks down over time and use: your car, house, television, computer, and even your body. If a particular "thing" is balanced and functioning correctly, it will predictably take much longer for it to break down. However, if it is imbalanced or its structure is poor, and it's not working correctly, it will break down faster. Your body is no different. If your body is not lined up properly, and is poorly balanced, physical, chemical, and emotional stress will cause your body to break down faster and be less healthy.

Dr. James Chestnut has a great analogy describing the interplay of stress and how it causes imbalances, which cause stress on your nerves, bones, ligaments, and muscles.

Imagine your body floating in water. On your arms, you have water wings with little holes where the air is slowly releasing. These water wings signify your lifespan, which is approximately 120 years with no stress on your body. You also have on a backpack. Every physical, chemical, or emotional stress you put onto or into your body is like a rock going into the backpack. Some rocks are bigger than others, like smoking, overeating, taking drugs, and having poor posture. The more and bigger rocks you have in the backpack, the more you are going to sink and struggle to keep afloat. The pressure around the water wings will increase, causing more air to come out, affecting your lifespan. The bad news is the more rocks you put into your backpack, the more you will struggle through life. The good news is you can take those rocks out of your backpack by taking part in healthy activities.

Poor Structure = Poor Function

If the structure of anything is poor, the function is going to be less than ideal. If your body's structure is poor, its function will suffer. The most important function that will suffer is its healing ability.

But from where does this healing come? The very first things to form when you were growing inside your mom's belly were your brain and spinal cord. The second structures to form were your skull and spine to protect them. Obviously, that shows you how important those organs and structures are. The brain is the master control center for every function in your body. For your lungs to breathe, heart to beat, stomach to digest, and intestines to absorb, the message has to come from the brain, down the spinal cord and through the nerves. The brain, spinal cord, and all the nerves are called your nervous system. The one thing that cannot be replaced in your body is your nervous system; therefore, it would be a good idea to take care of it.

If the bones of your spine are lined up as intended, your brain can send a signal down the spinal cord, and out to the rest of your body through the nerves. This allows your body to reach an optimal level of health. However, imbalances in your spine and posture can cause stress on the nerves exiting the spine, as well as on your bones, ligaments, and muscles. Stress over time leads to breakdown and symptoms.

It may be helpful to use a plumbing analogy to describe the nervous system. The brain is the faucet. The main hose is the spinal cord coming down from the brain. Connected to the main hose are numerous smaller hoses, which represent the nerves. Just like the hoses that deliver water to all parts of your lawn, the nerves send messages to every cell, tissue, and organ in your body.

Pain is not the best indicator that your body may be physically imbalanced. You can have an imbalance without even knowing it, while it is insidiously breaking down your body. Forty percent of nerve function is lost before you feel pain. Additionally, your nerves are so sensitive that the weight of a quarter causes a nerve to lose 50% of its function. Very rarely is a nerve pinched between two bones. Using the hose analogy, if you lose 50% of the water to your lawn, your grass will be fine for a day, a week, or maybe even a month. Over months, however, your grass will cease to grow without the appropriate water flow. If your body does not have the appropriate nerve flow because of an imbalance that has developed over time, your health will be damaged.

A common physical stress that can cause the first physical imbalance is something you probably would not even consider. It is something that happens very early in life, way too early for you to even remember. The birthing process! The delivery process is very traumatic, whether it is natural or through a C-section. Not only is it traumatic for the mother, but even more so for the baby. Its head, neck, and shoulders are twisted and turned, tractioned and depressed with a lot of force.

I have three little girls and watched them all being born. My oldest had the cord wrapped around her neck, so they used a vacuum device on her head to yank her out. My second little girl also had the cord around her neck, but they did not use the vacuum device. Once her head came out of the birth canal, the doctor grabbed under her skull, on her head and neck, and proceeded to yank her out. Thankfully, the umbilical cord was not around our third girl's neck, but the delivery process was similar to that of our second little girl.

The baby has to come out, but there are consequences to these deliveries. The head is compressed, neck twisted from side to side, neck pulled and shoulders depressed. Do you think that physical stress could cause the imbalances in the spine, putting pressure on the nervous system? Absolutely! Just as with adults, if those imbalances are present, over time more stress is placed on the nerves, bones, ligaments, and muscles, causing breakdown and symptoms. Some symptoms of these imbalances include colic, asthma-type symptoms, reflux-type symptoms, ear infections, frequent colds, and constipation. If there is interference in the communication between the brain and the organs, the body is not going to heal properly and symptoms will result. The sooner these imbalances are identified and corrected, the healthier the baby will be.

As a chiropractor, I identify imbalances in my patients' structure. I help to correct the posture, taking the pressure off the nerves, bones, ligaments, and muscles, thus allowing the body to heal. The time it takes to correct your structure depends on the time the stress has been on your body and the imbalances that develop. A newborn will be corrected much faster than an adult who has had more stress and imbalances in his body. In general, it could take anywhere from three months to two years to correct your structure, depending on your structural imbalances.

Action Steps to Achieving Physical Balance

1. **Identify any structural imbalances in your body.** To identify gross imbalance, simply look at yourself in the mirror. Is one shoulder higher than the other?

Is one hip higher than the other? Are your feet flat, in other words, pronated? Is one foot flatter than the other? Is one foot flared out more than the other? Are your knees rotated in or out? You can also see if your head is jutting out away from your body. Are your shoulders rolled forward? Is your low back arched too much or not enough? Is your mid back rounded excessively? Another test is a leg length check. Lie down on your stomach on your bed with your head straight and feet hanging off the end. Have somebody look to see if one leg is shorter than the other.

Balanced Structure

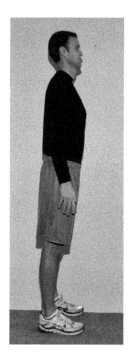

Head centered
over shoulders

Shoulders neutral

Mid back
slightly convex to
the back

Low back
slightly convex
to the front

Pelvis neutral

Hips neutral

Knees neutral

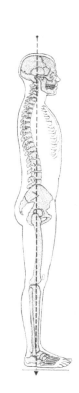

33

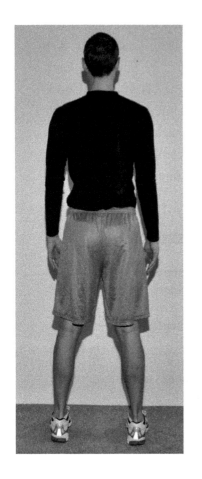

Head neutral
with no tilt or
rotation

Shoulders level

Mid back
straight

Low back
straight

Pelvis and hips
level

Knees straight,
not bowed or
knock-kneed

Feet parallel or
toed out
slightly;

Achilles tendon
straight

Ankles neutral

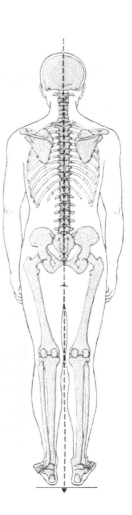

Imbalanced Structures

Kyphosis-Lordosis Posture

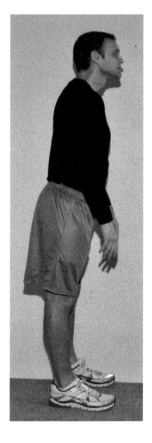

Head forward
from body

Shoulders
rolled forward

Mid back
excessively
rounded

Low back
excessively
arched

Pelvis
anteriorly
tilted

Hips flexed

Knees
hyperextended

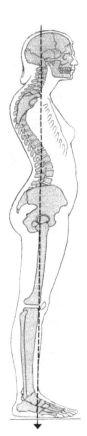

35

Sway Back Posture

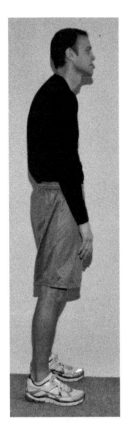

Head forward
from body

Shoulders rolled
forward

Mid back
excessively
rounded

Low back
flattened

Pelvis
posteriorly tilted

Hips pushed
forward

Knees
hyperextended

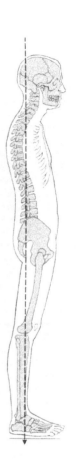

Crooked Man

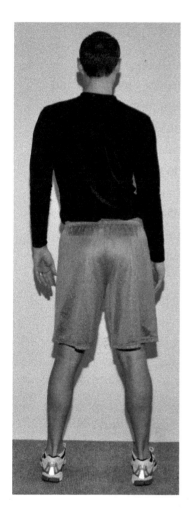

Head neutral with no tilt or rotation

Shoulders unlevel (left high)

Mid back deviated from center (to the left)

Low back deviated from center (to the left)

Pelvis unlevel (right high)

Hips deviated (to the right)

Knees bowed or knock-kneed (left rotated inward)

Feet flat or rolled inward (on left); Achilles tendon bowed

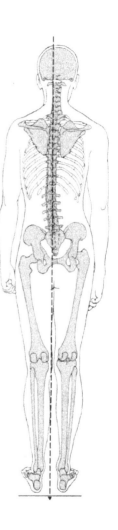

2. **Determine the weak or inflexible areas of your body.** My three favorite tests, which give a wealth of information, are the Overhead Deep Squat, Active

Straight Leg Raise, and Seated Rotation tests. These tests are all part of the Functional Movement Screen. To learn more about this screen, please go to www.FunctionalMovement.com.

The Overhead Deep Squat assesses mobility and stability of the entire body. To do a proper squat, you need full range of motion at all of your joints, as well as the core stability to coordinate and execute the movement against gravity. To do it, stand with your feet hip to shoulder width apart and parallel to each other. Your arms are held overhead with your elbows straight. Keep your heels on the floor and squat as low as possible, relatively slowly. Errors include your heels coming off the floor, feet flattening or rotating outward, knee(s) buckling inward, low back arching or rounding, pelvis deviating to one side, arms falling forward, elbows flexing, or neck hyperextending.

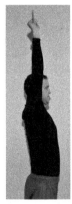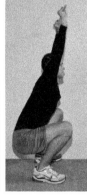

The Active Straight Leg Raise assesses hamstring flexibility in relation to core stability. This screen is performed actively (instead of passive flexibility assessment) to determine your true available range of motion. For example, it does not help you to have flexible hamstrings if you cannot use them without straining the stability of the core to get that range of motion. Lie on your back with both legs straight. Lift up one leg, keeping that ankle relaxed and the leg straight. The opposite thigh should remain still and straight. Normal range of motion is approximately 80 to 90 degrees. Perform three (3) reps on each side, observing when legs or pelvis are no longer still and stable. Errors include not lifting leg with knee straight to 80 to 90 degrees, elevating opposite thigh, and not keeping pelvis still.

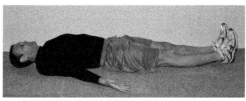

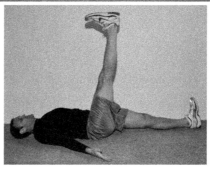

The Seated Rotation test assesses hip and spinal mobility in relation to core integrity and stability. This is a difficult posture and movement if your hips are restricted, core muscles are relatively weak, or thoracic spine mobility is restricted. Sit up tall with your legs crossed on the floor, and arms crossed in front of your chest. Rotate to each side. Normal range of motion (thoracic rotation) is approximately 45 degrees. Errors include difficulty staying upright, difficulty rotating to either side, or legs lifting off the floor.

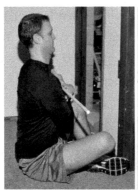 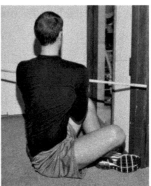

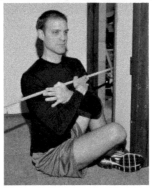

If you have weak or inflexible joints and muscles, you will not be able to do these tests properly.

3. **Consult with a trained professional like a wellness chiropractor, physical therapist, certified strength and conditioning specialist, or certified personal trainer.** Many know how to perform these tests to determine if anything is out of balance. An added advantage of a wellness chiropractor is their capability to take x-rays of your spine to see the internal structure. If your internal structure is poor, chances are your external function will be poor. The x-rays show what your spinal curves look like and are more accurate in assessing your posture. Additionally, x-rays show how stress is placed on your bones, nerves, muscles, and ligaments, and even how long the stress has been on your spine.

4. **Correct your structure.** Once you have identified the problem, it will not get any better unless you do things differently. Remember Albert Einstein's definition of insanity: doing the same thing repeatedly and expecting a different result. If you keep doing what you've always done, you'll always get what you've already got. Correction of your structure usually includes spinal adjustments, extremity adjustments, corrective exercises, nutritional supplements, orthotic supports, flexibility exercises, and strengthening exercises.

EXERCISE: LIFE IS MOVEMENT

NOWADAYS, WE HAVE AN ALARMING epidemic in the United States. One in three adults are obese. One in five children are overweight and likely to carry their health problems into adulthood. Twenty-one million people have diabetes. One in five adults have arthritis. In the United States, these types of conditions affect nearly 50% of the population and contribute to seven of every ten deaths.

Maybe you're wondering what is this crisis. It is the number one problem in the United States, and it is not the economy. It's chronic diseases and illnesses. Some examples are heart disease, cancer, diabetes, depression, chronic pain, obesity, and arthritis. These are all chronic, which means they have developed over time, but they are preventable.

- We spend a lot of money on healthcare in this country, but we do not get a lot in return. American healthcare and insurance use high-cost tests, procedures, and drugs to treat acute illness with less emphasis on wellness and prevention. In 2008, The

Center for Disease Control and Prevention stated, within its Budget Request Summary, how important it is to prevent chronic diseases, and how doing so would decrease healthcare spending. However, *less than three percent* of their 2008 budget was allocated toward chronic disease prevention. Here are some numbers that will shock you. In America, we spend the following amounts to diagnose and treat these diseases:

- $834,000,000 for heart disease (including coronary heart disease, congestive heart failure, part of hypertensive disease, cardiac dysrhythmias, rheumatic heart disease, cardiomyopathy, pulmonary heart disease, and other or ill-defined "heart" diseases)
- $209,000,000 for cancer
- $476,000,000 for diabetes
- $120,000,000 for depression
- $167,000,000 for chronic pain
- $350,000,000 for arthritis
- $320,000,000 for obesity

That's a lot of money, don't you think? Actually, those amounts are what is spent *per day, not per year,* on those diseases! These are preventable diseases. It's quite disheartening to accept the reality that we have become that unhealthy. The good news is you can prevent or at least reduce your chances of developing a chronic disease by incorporating simple lifestyle changes.

The causes of death in the United States are just as staggering as the money spent. For example, poor diet and physical inactivity kill over 7,000 people per week. If you think drugs are going to help you get healthy, think again. Reactions to prescription drugs kill over 600 people per week, while over-the-counter medications like aspirin, Tylenol, ibuprofen, and NSAIDs kill 146 people per week. Therefore, you have to make lifestyle changes if you want to get healthy, not just pop a pill. I want to help you develop beneficial lifelong habits that will help keep you healthy.

Simple Lifestyle Changes

Remember, these are simple, but not always easy. That is why we have developed these chronic health problems. These lifestyle changes are all geared to take physical, chemical, emotional, and mental stress away from your body.

These changes are:
1. Participate in moderate, regular exercise.
2. Incorporate healthier eating habits.
3. Align and balance your body.
4. Align and balance your mind.

Unfortunately, most healthcare practitioners fail to counsel their patients on these issues. I'm not your typical healthcare practitioner. I want to help you succeed in getting and staying healthy. Ask yourself these questions: Can I improve my own health? Can I take responsibility for my health? Do I want to take control of my health? Will I do the work necessary to become and stay healthy? If all your answers are "yes", you are on your way to a healthier life.

Roadblocks to Exercise

We all have roadblocks that prevent us from exercising. The first is the broad category of excuses. Some common ones are:

- You don't have time.
- You're too tired.
- You don't know what to do.
- You have to work.
- It's too hard.

You can overcome the excuses. The first way to overcome them is to examine your belief system. What have you learned about exercising over the years? Why do you think you can't exercise, or what is preventing you from being healthy? Too often, we equate exercise with pain. We have to reverse that. We have to equate exercise with health and all the benefits it produces. It increases your strength, mood, immune system function, self-esteem, brainpower, memory, bone density, and energy. Exercise decreases your risk of heart disease, cancer, high blood pressure, diabetes, obesity, osteoporosis, cholesterol, depression, and body fat. Connect exercise with how good it makes you feel, and that will make it much easier to exercise.

At an early age, you may have learned subconsciously that exercise is bad. This commonly happens in youth athletics, and my athletic career was no different. What happened in sports if you lost a game, didn't play hard, or made a mistake? The coaches would make you run laps, do pushups, or do some other physical activity as punishment. Never use exercise as punishment! That plants the seed that exercise is bad and eventually that seed will firmly root itself within you. Always connect rewards and positive consequences to exercise.

The second way is to determine why it is important for you to exercise. Finding your motivation will help you commit to exercise. Your motivation could be to live longer, live better, get rid of pain, lose weight, lower your blood pressure, or hundreds of other goals. These reasons help motivate you through the obstacles you will face in your daily life. As an example, my goals are to live as long and well as I can. I want to be active now with my children, and in the future with my grandchildren, great-grandchildren, and even my great-great-grandchildren. To do that, I have to incorporate exercise into my life *right now*, not in two, five, or ten years. If I don't practice healthy habits, how can I ask you to do it? Those are my goals, and they help motivate me through my daily obstacles.

Another good starting point is to determine your current fitness level. Get a physical, including your blood pressure, body fat percentage, and even a three-minute step test to determine where you are at the moment. Then, you can test yourself again in one month, two months, or three months, to see the improvement.

You can also list your favorite activities such as cardiovascular exercises, strength activities, flexibility exercises, walking the dog, biking, swimming, lifting weights, running, jogging, or participating in races. Next, schedule your exercise and keep your appointments. The last tip is one of my favorites, called the five-minute compromise. Exercise for five minutes, and if you don't feel like continuing, just stop. Most of the time you will keep going, but it is all right if you stop because you allowed yourself that compromise. You could even experiment and raise the compromise to eight or 10 minutes. Do not criticize yourself if you stop, because that will just cause more stress and unhealthy thinking.

Types of Exercise
Cardiovascular Training
These are activities that get your heart rate at or above 65% of your maximum heart rate, which is called your target heart rate, for 25 to 45 minutes. Your target heart rate is the pulse rate at which you will safely receive the maximum benefits. Examples of cardiovascular activities include biking, jogging, walking briskly, playing a sport, circuit training, swimming, using aerobic machines, and water aerobics.

To determine your target heart rate, calculate your maximum heart rate, which equals 220 minus your age.

47

Multiply your maximum heart rate by 65% and 90% to determine your target heart rate range to exercise in for 25 to 45 minutes, three to five days a week. This is an estimate, but is a very convenient and easy calculation.

An indirect measure of your target heart rate is your breathing rate. For example, if your breathing rate increases while you are exercising, but you can carry on a conversation, you're in the lower end of the range between 65% to 75%. If your breathing rate increases to a point at which you cannot carry on a conversation, you are in the upper range. When you're just starting, it is a good idea to start at a lower percentage, and as you get in better shape, increase your intensity toward the higher percentage. You may also alternate workouts into low, medium, and high intensity days.

Resistance Training
Resistance training is classically referred to as "lifting weights." This category includes any exercise that provides resistance such as calisthenics, body weight exercises, sit ups, pushups, pull ups, Pilates, Olympic lifting, power lifting, resistance/elastic bands, medicine balls, barbells, and dumbbells.

Resistance training helps you build muscle, increasing your lean body mass and decreasing your body fat. More muscle means you will burn more calories throughout the day, resulting in more fat loss. This type of exercise has definitely gained popularity with women over the last twenty years. It was commonly a missing link. Women would perform cardiovascular exercises like aerobics, but skip resistance training, because they thought they would get huge muscles, which will not happen.

It is important to integrate muscle and movement, and not to isolate muscles, with resistance training. That is, exercise multiple joints and muscles simultaneously. Your body was designed to move; therefore, when you train the movement you will move better and your muscles will get stronger. However, if you only focus on building the muscle, the movement may not improve. A prime example of training muscle and not movement is a body builder. A body builder trains the muscle to build it, but as a result becomes less mobile. The last benefit of integrating muscle and movement is efficiency. You will be able to perform a full workout in less time, and that is a definite advantage with our busy lives.

There are eight different movement patterns your body needs to learn. Following is each movement with example exercises, which train that movement.

1. Hip and Leg Pushing: Squats, Lunges, Step Ups
2. Hip Extension: Dead Lifts, Hip Lifts, Hip Hinge
3. Core Stabilization: Back Bridges, Side Bridges, Elbow Bridges
4. Rotation: Lying Trunk Twists, Medicine Ball Chops
5. Vertical Pulling: Chin Ups, Pull Ups, Cable or Elastic Band Pull Downs

6. Vertical Pushing: Dumbbell Shoulder and Military Presses
7. Horizontal Pulling: Bent Over Dumbbell Rows, Inverted Rows, Cable or Elastic Band Rows
8. Horizontal Pushing: Pushups, Dumbbell Chest Presses, Bench Presses

Mobility and Flexibility Training
Three different methods categorize Mobility and Flexibility training. First, active flexibility exercises actively take your body through ranges of motion to stretch and relax the muscles. Standing straight leg raises is an example. This type is best served during a warm up.

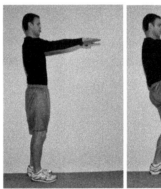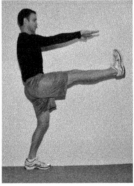

Swing one leg up and over shoulder height. Keep the leg straight during the swinging motion. Repeat with the opposite leg, attempting to swing the leg slightly higher with each repetition. Keep your trunk straight during the entire exercise.

Second, myofascial release, or a massage technique, loosens the muscles, relaxes the nerves, increases blood flow, and aids in recovery. A foam roll is a great tool that uses deep compression to roll out the muscle spasms that develop over time. The foam roll is an 18-inch long roll of tightly packed foam that about 5 inches in diameter. Even though you will probably enjoy the foam roll, there will be uncomfortable points during the routine. It will get easier and more comfortable after a few weeks, but at first it's going to hurt a little bit more. This is a good barometer of the tissue quality because the less it hurts, the higher the quality of tissue.

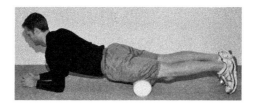

Foam Roll Quads. Lie with the roll under your quads. Roll the entire length of your quads from hips to knees. To create more compression, cross one leg over the other so only one leg is on the roll.

Myofascial release is important because it helps release the "knots" and spasms in the muscles. If you're just stretching, but you have these knots and spasms in the muscle, the muscle won't fully relax. Envision tying a knot in a string. The string will shorten, but if you just keep pulling at the ends, the knots just keeps getting tighter and the string stays the same length. If you loosen up the knot first, it comes out a lot easier, similar to myofascial release.

The last type is called static flexibility. This is the classic form of flexibility in which you maintain the stretch position against an object. This is best served as part of a cool down and injury treatment plan, not necessarily during a warm up. An example is the hamstring stretch that is shown below.

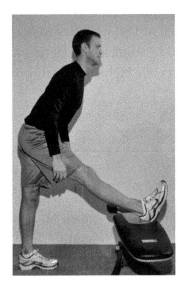

Place your heel or leg on object. Keep knee completely straight and toes pointed up. Keep your hips square and stance foot pointing directly forward or slightly in. Keep your back straight and slowly lean forward at hips until a stretch is felt in the back of your thigh.

Action Steps

1. **Determine your Target Heart Rate (THR).**
   Maximum Heart Rate (MHR) = 220 – your age = .
   beats per minute (bpm)

   THR = MHR x 0.65 = _____ bpm

   THR = MHR x 0.90 = _____ bpm

Keep your heart rate between these two numbers for 25-45 minutes 3-5 days/week.

2. **Learn these strength, balance, and mobility building exercises.**

HIP AND LEG PUSHING

Bodyweight Squat

1. Put your hands behind your neck.
2. Take your butt down and back (like you're going to sit on a chair).
3. Keep your knees over your toes and get your thighs parallel to the floor. Keep the weight of your body mostly toward your heels and make sure your heels stay down on the floor. Do not let your knees go in front of your toes.
4. When you come up, drive the heels into the floor.
5. If you can't perform correctly, keep your arms in front of you; this helps you keep your weight back. If you can't get your thighs to parallel, do ¼ or ½ squats.

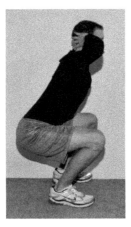 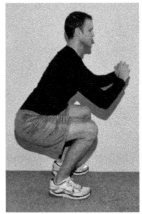

Split Squat

1. Take a long step forward with one leg.
2. Place your hands behind your head to keep your head and chest up (trunk straight).
3. Bend both knees as you drop the back knee down to the floor and keep the front knee over the foot.
4. Barely touch the back knee to the floor and push yourself up using mostly your front leg and repeat.
5. Repeat on other side.

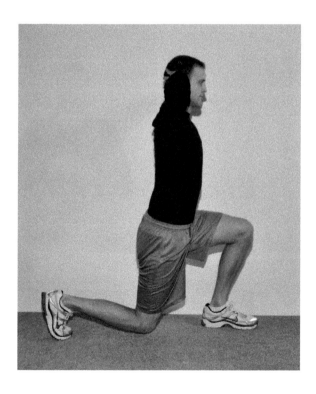

Side Squat

1. Stand with your feet approximately 4 feet apart and pointing straight ahead.
2. Sit to one side, taking your butt toward your leg.
3. Keep the weight on your heel as you sit down and back. Keep your knee over your toes.
4. Push yourself back up and repeat to the same side.
5. Then repeat the exercise on the other side.
6. A wider stance is better than a narrow stance for this exercise.

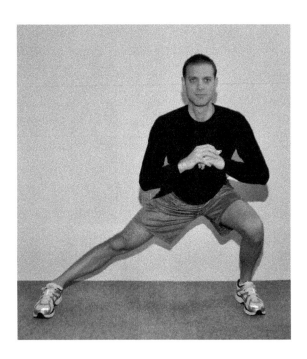

HIP EXTENSION

Hip Hinge

1. Stand with your feet about shoulder width apart.
2. Keep your back slightly arched, shoulder blades pulled back, and chest up.
3. While maintaining your back and knee position, bend from the hips and push the butt back (do not round your back).
4. Concentrate on pushing the butt back, not leaning forward. Your shoulders should remain over your toes.
5. *You should feel it in your hamstrings and glutes.* If you feel it more in your low back, you're doing it wrong.
6. To check yourself, hold a broomstick behind your back so it's touching your head and butt. If you're performing the hip hinge correctly, the stick will not lose contact with either your head or butt.
7. You can also stand so your back is facing the wall. When you perform the Hip Hinge, your butt should touch the wall.

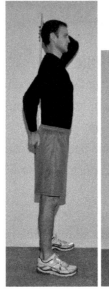 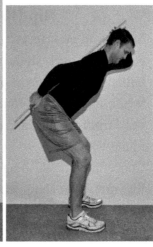

Start   Finish

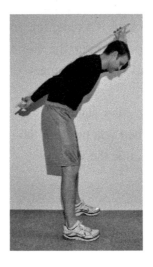

Incorrect

Single Leg Reach

1. Stand on one leg.
2. Reach out with both arms as you bend from your hip and let your other leg extend back. Keep your back straight; your body should form a straight line from head to heel.
3. Extend your stance hip and leg to return to the up position and repeat.
4. Repeat on the other leg.
5. Make sure you are reaching out, not just down in front of your feet.
6. You should feel this in your hips and thighs.

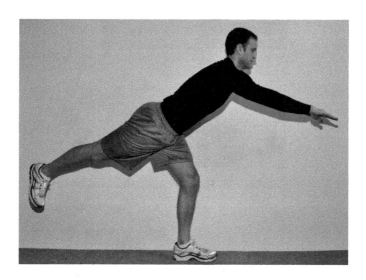

CORE STABILIZATION

Back Bridge

1. Lie on your back with your knees bent and feet flat on the floor (hook lying position).
2. Raise your hips to create a straight line from your knees to hips to shoulders.
3. Feel your glutes and hamstrings working, not the low back muscles.
4. Left your toes off the ground to target the glutes.

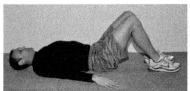

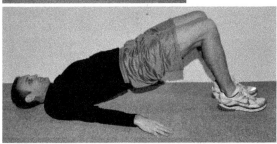

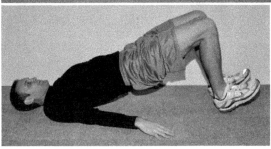

Elbow Bridge

1. Lie on your stomach.
2. Prop yourself up on your forearms so they are beneath your chest.
3. Lift your body off the floor forming a straight line from head to feet. Only your forearms and feet are touching the floor. Hold.
4. Keep your trunk straight and stable.
5. The further your arms are out in front of your body, the more difficult the exercise.

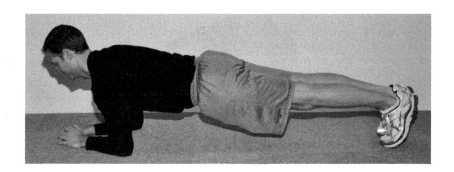

Bent Knee Side Bridge

1. Lie on your side with your knees bent. Form a straight line from your knees through your hips and to the shoulder.
2. With your weight supported on your forearm and hip/thigh, raise your hips/thighs off the floor so your weight is on your knee and lower leg. Hold.
3. Repeat on other side.
4. Maintain the straight line from shoulder to knees throughout the exercise.

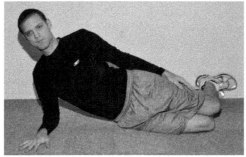

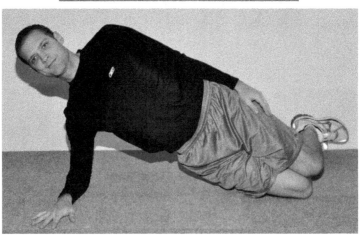

Straight Knee Side Bridge

1. Lie on your side so your entire body is in a straight line from head to heels.
2. Raise your body off the floor and hold.
3. Repeat on other side. When you perform this bridge only your forearm and foot are touching the ground.

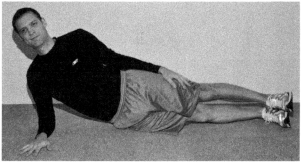

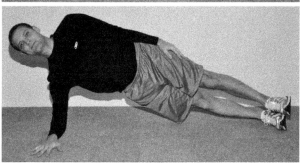

CORE ROTATION

Medicine Ball Hip Chops

1. Stand with a medicine ball in both hands. Put the ball next to your right hip.
2. Take the ball up and across your body like you're going to throw it over your left shoulder. Make sure to pivot on your right foot.
3. Bring it back down to your right hip and repeat.
4. Progressively increase the tempo of the chops (i.e. try to perform them faster and more powerfully).
5. Repeat from the left hip.
6. *If you don't have a medicine ball, use a dumbbell, another small weight, or nothing at all.*

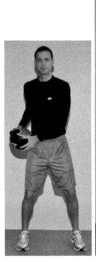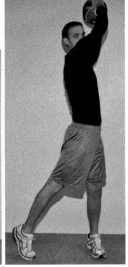

Medicine Ball Knee Chops

1. Stand with a medicine ball in both hands. Squat down and put the ball next to your right knee.

2. Take the ball up and across your body like you're going to throw it over your left shoulder. Make sure to pivot on your right foot.

3. Bring it back down to your right knee and repeat.

4. Progressively increase the tempo of the chops (i.e. try to perform them faster and more powerfully).

5. Repeat from the left knee.

6. *If you don't have a medicine ball, use a dumbbell, another small weight, or nothing at all.*

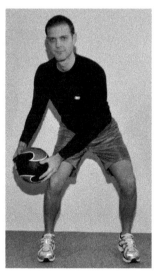 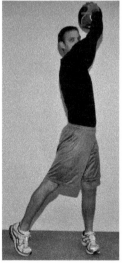

Medicine Ball Ankle Chops

1. Stand with a medicine ball in both hands. Squat down and put the ball next to your right ankle.
2. Take the ball up and across your body like you're going to throw it over your left shoulder. Make sure to pivot on your right foot.
3. Bring it back down to your right ankle and repeat.
4. Progressively increase the tempo of the chops (i.e. try to perform them faster and more powerfully).
5. Repeat from the left ankle.
6. *If you don't have a medicine ball, use a dumbbell, another small weight, or nothing at all.*

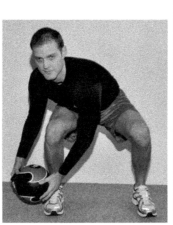 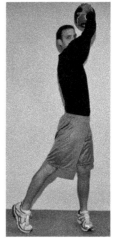

<u>VERTICAL PUSHING</u>

Dumbbell Shoulder Press

1. Stand with a dumbbell in each hand and raise them to your shoulders.
2. Keep the palms of your hands facing in toward your head and raise the dumbbells over your head.
3. Lower and repeat.

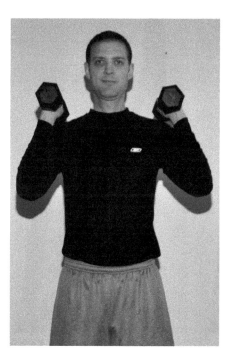
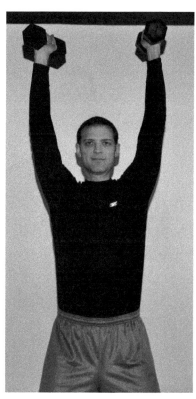

1 Arm Dumbbell Shoulder Press

1. Stand with a dumbbell in each hand and raise one to your shoulder.
2. Keep the palm of your hand facing in toward your head and raise the dumbbell over your head. Lower and repeat.
3. Repeat on the other side.

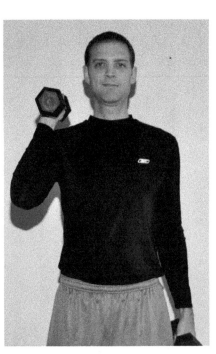
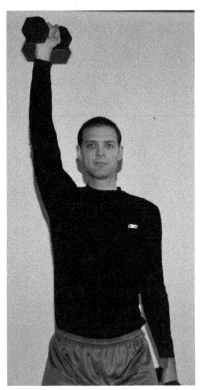

VERTICAL PULLING

*** If you cannot perform the Chin or Pull Ups, use the
assisted pull up machines at the gym, use a step to get
in the up position, and lower yourself down slowly, or
perform pulldowns using an elastic band or cable
pulley machine.**

Chin Ups

1. Grasp the bar with your palms facing your body.
2. Focus on pulling your elbows to your sides to
   pull your head above the bar.
3. Lower and repeat.

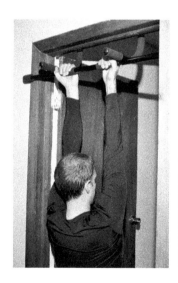
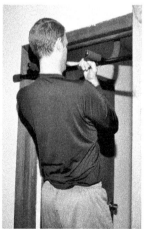

Parallel Grip Pull Ups

1. Grasp the bar with your palms facing each other.
2. Focus on pulling your elbows to your sides to pull your head above the bar.
3. Lower and repeat.

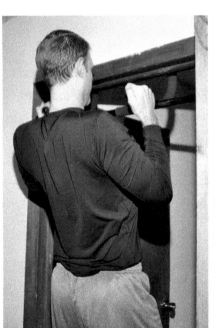 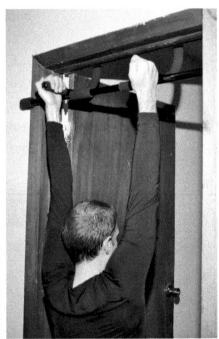

Pull Ups

1. Grasp the bar with your palms facing away from your body.
2. Focus on pulling your elbows to your sides to pull your head above the bar.
3. Lower and repeat.

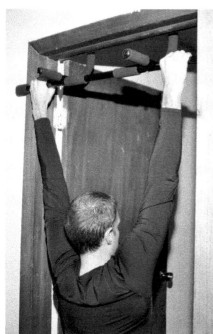
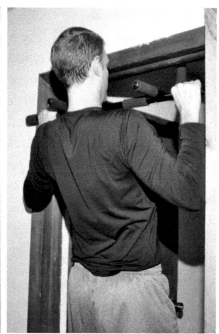

HORIZONTAL PUSHING

Pushups

1. Lie on your stomach with your toes on the ground and hands on the ground next to your shoulders.

2. Keep your body in a straight line while pushing your body away from the ground with your hands.

3. Lower and take your chest toward the ground. Push up and repeat.

4. Make sure your shoulders do not go below your elbows in the lowering phase. Keep your body in a straight line during the entire exercise without allowing your back to arch or round.

5. *If you cannot perform this correctly, perform them with your knees on the ground instead of your feet, with your hands elevated, or on a wall.*

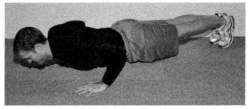

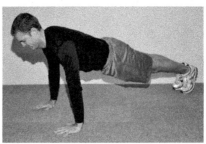

Hands Elevated Pushups

1. This is the same as regular pushups but now you will place your hands on a 12 (Low) to 48 (High) inch elevation. Stairs are a great place to perform this exercise.

2. Keep your body in a straight line with your arms outstretched. Lower and take your chest toward the elevation. Push up and repeat.

3. Make sure your shoulders do not go below your elbows in the lowering phase. Keep your body in a straight line during the entire exercise without allowing your back to arch or round.

4. *If this is too difficult, do the pushup with your hands on a wall.*

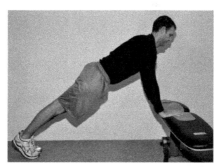

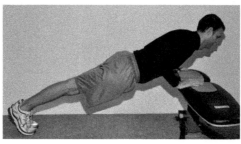

Wall Pushups

1. Stand with your feet two to four feet away from a wall. Place your hands on the wall slightly below shoulder level.

2. Keep your body in a straight line with your arms outstretched. Lower and take your chest toward the wall. Push away and repeat.

3. Make sure your shoulders do not go below your elbows in the lowering phase. Keep your body in a straight line during the entire exercise without allowing your back to arch or round.

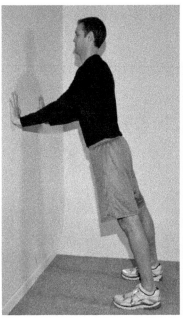
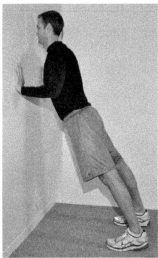

Dumbbell Bench Press

1. Lie on your back on a bench.
2. Hold the dumbbells at the outside edges of your shoulders, palms facing your thighs.
3. Lift both dumbbells straight over your chest. Lower them toward your shoulders but DO NOT go past the shoulders.
4. Lift them back over your chest and repeat.

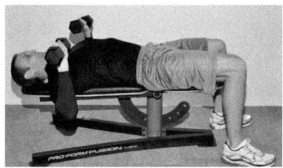

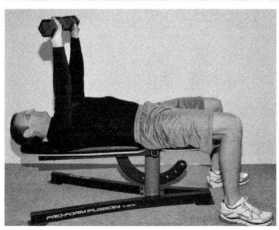

Alternating Dumbbell Bench Press

1. Lie on your back on a bench.
2. Hold the dumbbells at the outside edges of your shoulders, palms facing your thighs.
3. Alternate lifting the dumbbells, going back and forth between your right and left arms.
4. Lower each toward your shoulder but DO NOT go past the shoulder.

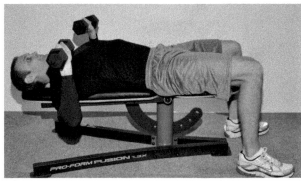

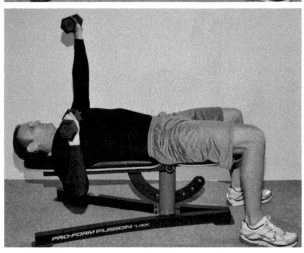

HORIZONTAL PULLING

Bench Dumbbell Row (Unsupported)

1. Get a wide stance with your knees over your feet.
2. Lean forward and place one hand on a bench. Keep your back straight and low back slightly arched.
3. Concentrate on first moving the shoulder blade back and then the elbow to bring the dumbbell to your side. Lower and repeat.
4. Repeat on other side.
5. Keep back straight during the entire exercise.

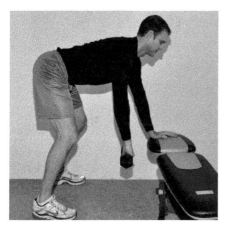 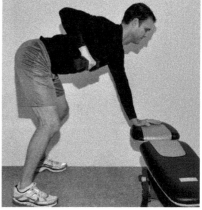

Bench Dumbbell Row (Supported)

1. Place one hand and knee on a bench. Hold a dumbbell in your other hand, hanging down.
2. Concentrate on first moving the shoulder blade back and then the elbow to bring the dumbbell to your side. Lower and repeat.
3. Repeat on other side.
4. Keep back straight during the entire exercise.

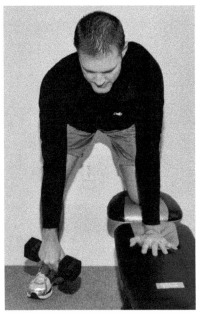
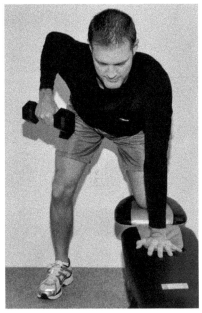

Inverted Row

1. Place a bar in a power rack or Smith machine at waist level.
2. Lie on your back with your chest under the bar and feet (heels) on the ground.
3. Grasp the bar with an overhand grip a little more than shoulder width apart.
4. Keep your body straight and pull your chest to the bar. Lower and repeat.
5. This exercise is basically a horizontal pull up.
6. *If you cannot perform at least 5 reps, bend your knees and place your feet flat on the floor or raise the bar higher in the rack.*

3. **Rest, Recover, Regenerate using the Foam Roll.** When using the foam roll, find a tender spot in the area you are working and keep the roll on this spot for 20 seconds or until the discomfort decreases by 50-75% (whichever comes first). Find other sensitive areas and repeat. Continue rolling regularly to keep the area relaxed after the area is free from pain. You should also experiment to see what position works best for you. You can purchase a foam roll at numerous sporting goods stores.

Foam Roll Calves

1. Sit with the roll under your calves.
2. Roll the entire length of your calves from knees to ankles.
3. To create more compression, cross one leg over the other so all the weight is on one leg.

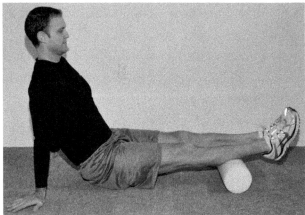

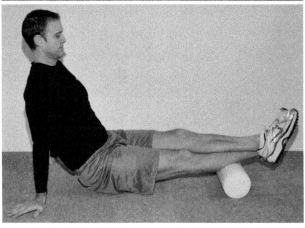

Foam Roll Hamstrings

1. Sit with the roll under your hamstrings.
2. Roll the entire length of your hamstrings from hips to knees.
3. To create more compression, cross one leg over the other so all the weight is on one leg.

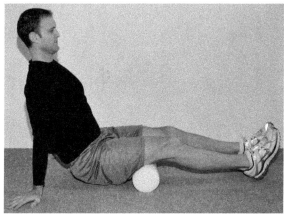

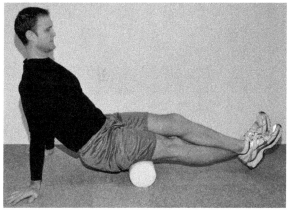

Foam Roll Glute & Piriformis

1. Sit on the roll and place your right ankle on your left knee.
2. Shift your body so your right glute is on the roll.
3. Roll back and forth over the hip area.
4. Repeat on other side.

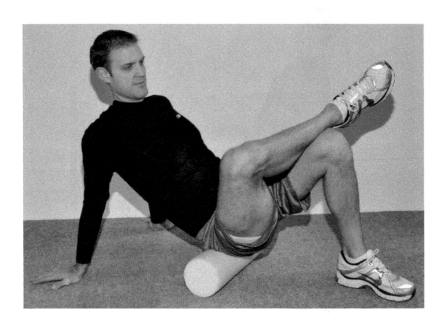

Foam Roll TFL & IT Band (Outer Thigh)

1. Lie on your side with the roll under your hip. Cross your top leg over your bottom leg.
2. Roll toward your knee and then back up to the hip.
3. Repeat on the other side.
4. To create more compression, stack your top leg onto your bottom leg.

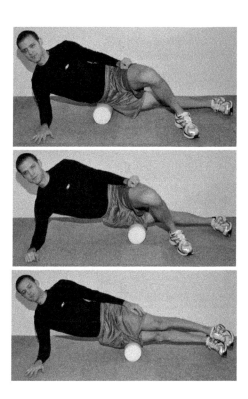

Foam Roll Quads

1. Lie with the roll under your quads.
2. Roll the entire length of your quads from hips to knees.
3. To create more compression, cross one leg over the other so all the weight is on one leg.

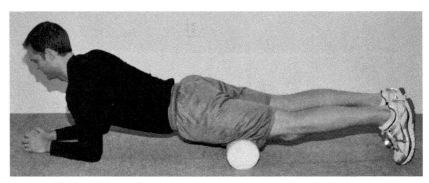

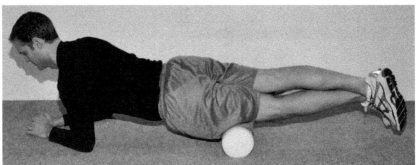

Foam Roll Adductors (Inner Thigh)

1. Lie with the roll under your adductors (inner thigh) on one leg.
2. Roll the entire length of your inner thigh from hips to knees.
3. Repeat on other side.

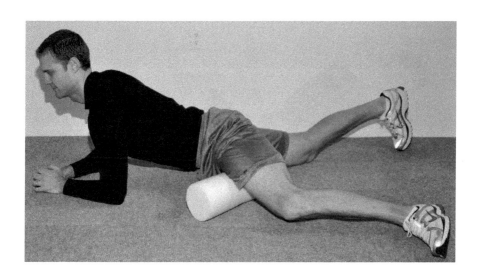

Foam Roll QL

1. Lie on your side with the roll under your low back.
2. Roll up and down over your low back.
3. Repeat on other side.

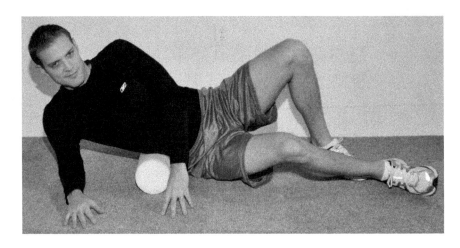

Foam Roll Lats

1. Lie on one side with the roll under your armpit.
2. Roll up and down the lat.
3. Repeat on the other side.

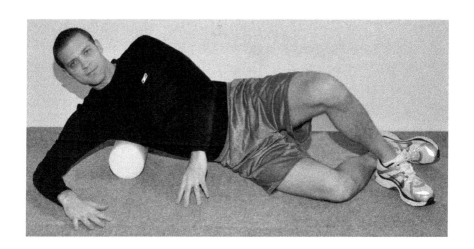

Foam Roll Spine

1. Lie with the roll under your lower mid back. Cross your arms over your chest.
2. Roll up to your upper back, then down again.
3. Repeat.
4. If your neck gets tired, place your hands behind your head and neck for support.

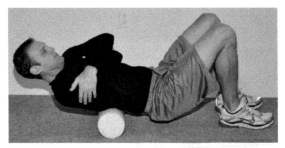

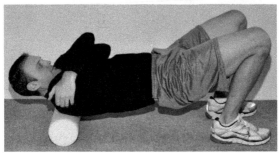

4. **Stretch your tight muscles.** There are muscles that are commonly tight in most individuals. Moreover, there are muscles that are prone to tightness, so it is important to stretch these muscles. When performing these stretches, hold the stretch for 25 to 30 seconds. It should be uncomfortable, but not painful.

Hamstring Stretch

1. Place your heel or leg on object. Keep knee completely straight and toes pointed up.
2. Keep your hips square and stance foot pointing directly forward or slightly in.
3. Keep your back straight and slowly lean forward at hips until a stretch is felt in the back of your thigh.
4. Repeat on other side.

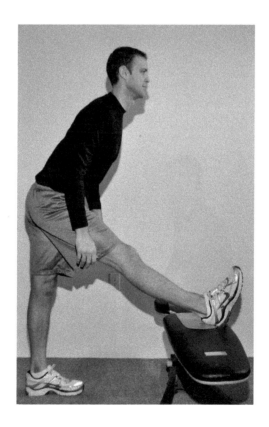

Sitting 90 90 Hip Stretch

1. Sit on the floor with one leg in front of you so your knee forms a 90 degree angle. Line up your knee to your shoulder.
2. Place the other leg behind you with that knee at a 90 degree angle.
3. With your shoulder and knee lined up, take your chest in the direction of your shin by bending at your hips.
4. You should feel a stretch in your hip and glute.
5. Repeat on the other side.

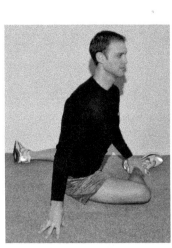
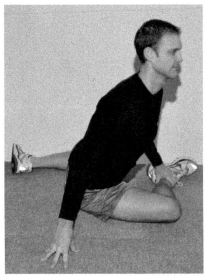

Kneeling Hip Flexor Stretch

1. Place your left knee on the ground at a 45 degree angle inward to an 18 to 24 inch elevation.
2. Bend your right leg and knee to place your right foot on the elevation in line with your left knee.
3. Keep your trunk upright as you lunge forward over the elevation.
4. Feel the stretch in the front of your left hip.
5. Do not let your back arch.
6. To increase the stretch, tuck your hips under slightly (the opposite of arching your back) and reach up with your left arm.
7. Repeat on the other side.

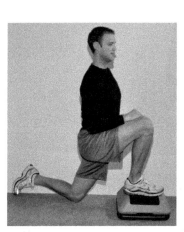
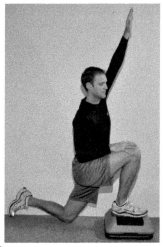

Sitting Adductor Stretch

1. Sit in front of a wall with your legs spread as much as possible.
2. Take your chest forward by bending from the hips.
3. Keep your trunk straight.
4. Feel the stretch in your inner thigh muscles.
5. You can also do this as a partner stretch instead of using a wall.

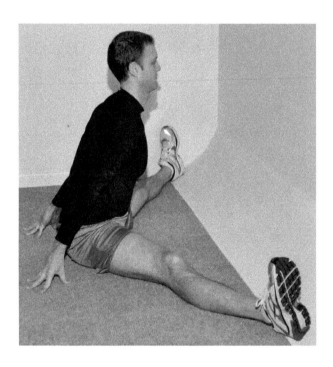

Kneeling Quad Stretch

1. Place your knees as close to a wall as possible.
2. Place the top of your left foot on the wall and your right foot on the ground in front of you.
3. Straighten your trunk.
4. Feel a stretch in the front of your left thigh, maybe even into the left front hip.
5. To increase the stretch, tuck your hips under slightly (the opposite of arching your back) and reach up with your left arm.
6. The goal is to have your lower leg parallel to the wall with the heel touching your glute. If you cannot do this, increase the distance from the wall until you become more flexible.
7. Repeat on the other side.

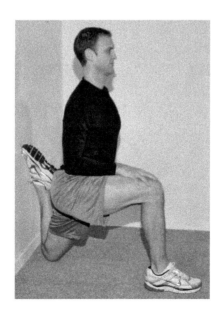

Kneeling Side Trunk Stretch

1. Kneel down and take your hips to your feet.
2. Take your chest toward the floor as you reach out in front of your body.
3. Walk your hands over to one side until you feel a stretch in the side of your trunk.
4. Hold.
5. Walk your hands over to the other side and hold.

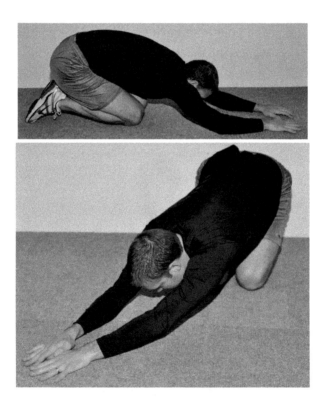

Doorway Pec Stretch

1. Stand with your forearms inside a doorway. Your elbows should be at shoulder level.
2. Step forward with one leg.
3. Lean forward until stretch is felt across chest.
4. You can also perform the stretch with your hands on the doorway at shoulder level. Your elbows should be relaxed as you lean forward.

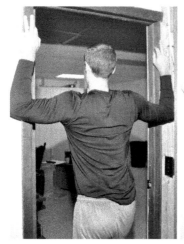 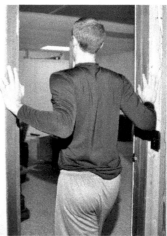

For more exercise programs, workouts, and videos, please go to www.TotalHealth-Fitness.com and become a Total Health Member for free.

NUTRITION BASICS: PRO-INFLAMMATION VS. ANTI-INFLAMMATION

IF YOU IMPROVE YOUR HEALTH, your symptoms will go away. Better yet, you may not even get symptoms. When you eat a pro-inflammatory diet, you are putting yourself at risk for more symptoms and diseases. You need to decide, even if you feel great, if you want to risk eating pro-inflammatory foods that can cause significant chronic diseases and health problems.

Pro-inflammatory foods include the following:

- "White" processed foods like enriched white bread, pasta, rice, bagels, pretzels, chips, crackers, and most packaged goods.
- Partially hydrogenated oils (trans fats) found in margarine, deep fried foods, and most packaged foods.
- Corn oil, safflower oil, sunflower oil, cottonseed oil, and soybean oil which are in mayonnaise, tartar

sauce, margarine, salad dressings, and many packaged foods.

- Soda (diet and regular), energy drinks, sugar.
- Meat and eggs from grain fed animals.

**Foods that fight inflammation
(i.e. anti-inflammatory) include the following:**

- Raw fruits and vegetables.
- Red and sweet potatoes.
- Fresh fish.
- Meat, chicken, and eggs from grass-fed animals. If you can't get these, get lean cuts of regular meat.
- Omega-3 eggs.
- Raw nuts like almonds, walnuts, and cashews.
- Spices: ginger, turmeric, garlic, dill, oregano, coriander, fennel, red chili pepper, basil, and rosemary.
- Organic extra virgin olive oil and coconut oil. Butter is much better than margarine.
- Use extra virgin olive oil, balsamic vinegar, lemon juice or mustard for salad dressing.
- Drink water and organic green tea. Red wine and stout beer are the best choices if you choose to drink.
- Dark chocolate for your sweet tooth.

Because our diets are filled with pro-inflammatory foods, it is also important to add nutritional supplements into your health plan. A high quality multivitamin &

multimineral supplement, antioxidants, and Omega-3 fish oil are essential to a well-rounded wellness program.

Do We Need Carbohydrates?

With many diets touting the bad effects of carbohydrates, you may think the answer is no. However, in reality, WE NEED THEM! Carbohydrates are made of simple and complex sugars, starches, and fibers. They play a role in the structure and function of your cells and organs, and provide energy for the body. They provide us with vitamins, minerals, phytochemicals, fiber, and energy for the brain and nervous system.

There are good and bad sources of carbohydrates. Because of the convenience factor, many people get their carbohydrates from bad sources. They usually come in pre-packaged foods, including refined cereals, white bread and flour, crackers, cookies, chips, doughnuts, soda, and many others. These are refined, which means they are stripped of the vitamins, minerals, phytochemicals, and fiber that we need. Good sources are unrefined carbohydrates, such as whole fruits, vegetables, and whole grains.

Carbohydrates fall under scrutiny because we tend to overindulge in the wrong kinds, usually all at once. This causes blood glucose to rise rapidly, releasing more insulin than is needed to take the glucose into the cells. With too much insulin, the blood glucose levels plummet. The brain feels deprived of food and signals for more energy. This usually results in consuming more carbohydrates, which the body does not need at that time. Ingesting more unrefined carbohydrates stimulates more insulin production and creates an undesirable cycle.

Shopping List for Good Carbohydrates

Vegetables

Asparagus	Red Peppers	Broccoli
Mushrooms	Yellow Peppers	Spinach
Zucchini	Green Peppers	Kale
Cucumbers	Onions	Cabbage
Green beans	Peas	Romaine lettuce
Brussels sprouts	Corn	Yams
Carrots	Red potatoes	
Celery		

Fruits

Apples	Apricots	Berries (straw-,
Nectarines	Cherries	blue-, black-,
Peaches	Dates	rasp-)
Kiwi	Grapes	Cantaloupe
Grapefruit	Bananas	Watermelon
Oranges		

Cereals and Grains

Black beans	Rye bread	**Avoid white
Garbanzo beams	Cereals	flour
Whole grain	(with short list	("enriched"),

bread	of ingredients)	bagels, processed
(whole wheat		foods, pastas,
flour)		tortillas, etc

Avoid

Partially hydrogenated soybean oil

High fructose corn syrup

Sugar and artificial sweeteners (Splenda, Equal) – use

Agave syrup or cane sugar

What Is Protein?

Protein is another essential component to total health nutrition. Proteins build muscle, create hormones, transport vitamins, and maintain blood, skin, immune system, and connective tissue. They are made up of amino acids. You need a total of twenty-two amino acids. Your body makes thirteen of them, so nine are brought into your body through your diet. These nine are called essential amino acids.

There are two different types of protein. First, there are complete proteins. These contain all nine of the essential amino acids and come from animal sources like meat, fish, poultry, and eggs. The second type is incomplete proteins, which are missing one or two of the essential amino acids. These come from plant sources like beans, peas, nuts, and seeds. If you are a vegetarian, you need to eat various sources of protein to ensure you receive all the essential amino acids.

Shopping List for Protein

Meat
Skinless boneless chicken breast
Skinless boneless turkey breast
Lean pork
Flank steak
Venison
Buffalo

Fish
Salmon (preferably organic)
Tuna
Cod (preferably organic)
Shrimp

Eggs and Dairy
Free range eggs
Organic cheese
Organic yogurt
Organic skim milk

Soy
Nuts
Tofu
Beans

Protein Powders
Whey
- Concentrate: lower processing, lower protein

- Isolate: high processing, higher protein
- Hydrolyzed: Predigested by enzymes so it can enter the blood faster. This is good if it is taken up by the muscles, but bad if it's not.

Casein
- Main protein in milk. Releases the amino acids slower into the blood so there is a steady flow.

**It is ideal to combine the whey and casein for optimal protein.

Is Fat Bad?

We Americans are obsessed with "low fat" or "non fat" foods. The truth is, fat is good for you! Here are a few reasons:

- Essential for body energy and cell growth.
- Helps absorb nutrients.
- Protects organs, especially your BRAIN!
- Keeps your body warm.
- Helps to produce important hormones.
- Decreases the desire to overeat.

Obviously, some fats are better than others. Omega-3 and Omega-9 fatty acids are your best choices, while you want to limit or avoid trans, saturated, and Omega-6 fatty acids as much as possible. The problem for Americans is that we consume too many of the trans, saturated, and Omega-6 fats. The health benefits of eating good fats include:

Decreases	Improves
Inflammation	Immune system function
Arthritis symptoms	Brain development, focus
Cancer incidence	Cognitive skills
Migraine headaches	Skin, hair, nails
Post-menopausal symptoms	Absorption of vitamins
Depression	Weight loss
Constipation	Body temperature regulation
High blood pressure	Cardiovascular health
Cholesterol	Hormonal balance
Platelet aggregation	Overall health and well being
	ADHD

Taken from *Chris Johnson's Meal Patterning*

Shopping List for Fat

Trans Fatty Acids (avoid as much as possible)
Hydrogenated and partially hydrogenated oils
Margarine (use butter instead)
Shortening

Saturated Fatty Acids (avoid as much as possible)
Butter
Palm kernel oil
Coconut oil

Omega-9 Fatty Acids (Monounsaturated)
Canola mayo

Extra virgin olive oil
Expeller pressed canola oil
Olives
Avocados
Natural peanut butter
Almonds
Almond butter
High oleic expeller pressed safflower or sunflower oil
Cashews
Hazelnuts
Macadamia nuts

Omega-6 Fatty Acids (limit these)

Evening primrose oil
Borage oil
Pumpkin seed oil
Soybean oil
Sesame seed oil

Omega-3 Fatty Acids (Polyunsaturated)

Flaxmeal
Flaxseed oil
Fish oils
Walnuts

How to Use and Understand
the Nutrition Facts Label

Nutrition Facts	
Serving Size 1 cup (228 g)	
Serving Per Container 2	
Amount Per Serving	
Calories 250 Calories from Fat 110	
	% Daily Value
Total Fat 12 g	18%
Saturated Fat 3 g	15%
Trans Fat 3 g	
Cholesterol 30 mg	10%
Sodium 470 mg	20%
Total Carbohydrate 31 g	10%
Dietary Fiber 0 g	0%
Sugars 5 g	
Protein 5 g	
Vitamin A	4%
Vitamin C	2%
Calcium	20%
Iron	4%

% Daily Values are based on a 2,000 calorie diet. Your Daily Values may be higher or lower depending on your calorie needs.

	Calories: 2,000	2,500
Total Fat	Less Than 65g	80 g
Sat Fat	Less Than 20 g	25 g
Cholesterol	Less Than 300 mg	300 mg
Sodium	Less Than 2,400 mg	2,400 mg
Total Carbohydrate	300 g	375 g
Dietary Fiber	25 g	30 g

1. **Start Here**
2. **Check Calories**
3. **Limit these nutrients**
4. **Get enough of these nutrients including fiber**
5. **Footnote**

105

1. The **Serving Size** is standardized to make it easier to compare similar foods. It is provided in familiar units, such as cups or pieces, followed by the metric amount, for example the number of grams.

2. **Calories and Calories from Fat** are a measure of how much energy you get from a serving of this food. Many Americans consume more calories than they need without meeting recommended intakes. **Remember: the number of servings you consume determines the number of calories you actually eat (your portion amount).**

3. **Limit the nutrients in #3**, most Americans get these in adequate amounts, or even too much. Eating too much fat, saturated fat, *trans* fat, cholesterol, or sodium may increase your risk of certain chronic diseases, like heart disease, some cancers, or high blood pressure.

4. Most Americans don't get enough dietary fiber, vitamin A, vitamin C, calcium, and iron in their diets. Eating enough of these nutrients can improve your health and help reduce the risk of some diseases and conditions.

5. The **Footnote** is always the same. It doesn't change from product to product because it shows recommended dietary advice for all Americans — it is not about a specific food product.

6. The **Percent Daily Value (%DV)** is based on the Daily Value recommendations for key nutrients but only for a 2,000 calorie diet — not 2,500 calories. You, like most people, may not know how many calories you consume in a day. However, you can still use the %DV as a frame of reference whether or not you consume more or less than 2,000 calories. **5%DV or less is low and 20% DV or more is high.**

7. "Ingredients" is not shown on this label but may be the most important aspect. In general, the more ingredients you see, the unhealthier it is for your body.

Action Steps

1. **Substitute an Unhealthy Version with the Healthy Version.** Below you will find a list of foods to avoid and their healthy alternative:

Avoid	Healthier Choice
Fried Foods (chicken, fish, etc.)	Baked or Grilled Foods
Soda pop (diet or regular) If you're going to have soda, the regular version is actually "healthier" than diet.	Water or Natural Juices

Artificial Sweeteners (Equal, Splenda, Stevia)	Sugar or better yet, Agave syrup or Cane sugar
Margarine	Butter
Enriched White Flour (bread, rice, pasta)	Whole Wheat Flour
Fat Free Food (cheese, sour cream)	Regular Version
Regular Peanut Butter	Natural Peanut Butter
High Fructose Corn Syrup	Agave syrup or Cane sugar
Creamy Dressings	Vinaigrettes or Olive Oils
Coffee	Green Tea

2. Healthy Eating Starts with Healthy Grocery Shopping. Be prepared when you go to the store by making a list, planning meals ahead of time, and eating before going into the store. Shop the outer perimeter because that is where you will find the fruits, vegetables, dairy, meat, eggs, and organic section (usually). You can also

"Rainbow Shop" which means try to get every color of the rainbow in you cart (and I don't mean different colored boxes). Different colors equal a variety of nutrients.

3. **The 10 Power Foods.**
   1) **Almonds** - Magnesium, healthy fats, riboflavin
   2) **Apples** - Fiber, vitamin C, antioxidants
   3) **Berries** - Fiber, vitamins C & K, manganese
   4) **Broccoli** - Calcium, iron
   5) **Red Beans** - Fiber, Vitamin B6, energy!
   6) **Salmon** - Omega 3, protein
   7) **Spinach** - Iron, vitamins A & C, and folate
   8) **Avocados** - Vitamins C, E, & B6, potassium, fiber
   9) **Pomegranates** - Vitamin C, antioxidants, potassium
   10) **Wheat Germ** - Protein, fat, some fiber

4. **Go Organic.** Organic produce and foods are grown without added pesticides or fertilizers, which can contaminate the food. You can shop a local farmer's market or an open air market. There are also services that deliver organic goods to your house. In our area, it is called Door to Door Organics (www.doortodoororganics.com). If they are not in your area, you may find something similar where you live. Eatwild.com is also an excellent resource.

5. **Make the most of your mealtime.** First, you may have heard that breakfast is the most important meal of the day. It is. If you do not eat breakfast, you are putting your body in a mini-starvation state so it conserves body fat instead of breaking it down. Breakfast gets your metabolism cranking.

Second, eat five or six meals a day, not three. The concept is to eat *before* you get hungry. You will be less likely to overeat because you will snack throughout the day so you will not feel the need to gorge. Here is a simple plan to do it and the calories you will ingest:

Time	Calories
6:30a.m.	350
9:30a.m.	250
Noon	450
3:00p.m.	200
6:00p.m.	600
8:00p.m.	150
Total	**2000**

6. **3-Step Plan for Eating Out.** First, choose a restaurant that has fresh ingredients. You cannot control what ingredients the restaurant uses, but you can control how much you put into your mouth. Second, order from the appetizer menu,

110

but avoid fried foods. This step is tricky since there are many fried foods on the appetizer menu. Third, and most importantly, split an entrée with your dining companion or get a to-go box with your food order and put half of your order in the box as soon as your food comes.

7. **Take Nutritional Supplements Everyday.** This is a controversial topic. Some experts think that if you eat a healthy diet, you will get all the vitamins and minerals you need. Other experts report that because most Americans do not eat a healthy diet, you need to take additional vitamins and minerals. And yet another group says that even if you eat a healthy diet, you still are not getting adequate amounts of all the vitamins and minerals. I fall in all of these groups. At a minimum, you need to take a high quality multivitamin and multimineral supplement everyday. If you want even more benefit, there are three more supplements you should take every day: Omega-3 fish oils, antioxidants, and probiotics.

Omega-3 fish oils have been shown to decrease the risk of cardiovascular disease, cancer, depression, kidney disease, painful joints, and other inflammatory conditions. When you choose an Omega-3 fish oil supplement, make sure it has eicosapentaenoic acid (EPA) and docosahexaenoic acid (DHA) and does not say "concentrated." Antioxidants help neutralize free radicals, maximizing the body's ability to maintain health. This antioxidant activity supports energy levels and maintains optimal joint and cardiovascular health. Lastly, probiotics replenish the essential enzymes and "good" bacteria necessary for maximum absorption of nutrients. Though processed foods are convenient, they can hinder your body's ability to efficiently digest and reap the nutritional compounds necessary for health. In other words, these supplements make your body work better, that is, get healthy!

MENTAL BALANCE AND ALIGNMENT: DE-STRESS, NOT DISTRESS

REMEMBER THE THREE STRESSES that cause your body to get out of balance -- which creates pressure on your nervous system, bones, ligaments, and muscles -- and causes your body to work harder, break down, and cause pain and other symptoms? Mental and emotional stress is often forgotten as one of these potential dangers. It's ironic, considering it may be the most powerful stress. Many times, it is insidious; you don't know it's causing physical symptoms until it's too late. You may think it has no affect because there is nothing physically happening to your body.

When you have mental stress, you create reactions in the body, which send messages that request your attention. You might get indigestion, ulcers, headaches, high blood pressure, or some other symptoms that range from mild discomfort to serious illness. Because it takes time for these symptoms to occur, you may be confused about why you have physical symptoms in the first place. To counteract mental and emotional stress, we have to manage the stress to create mental balance and alignment.

Thoughts Turn into Things

The term "positive thinking" gets thrown around a lot. I used to think it was all a bunch of garbage. Yet the more I learned and actually thought about it, the more sense it made. If what you tell yourself day after day is negative, you will have negative results. Just the process of thinking negatively causes stress, but the negative results cause even more stress. Everything you do starts with a thought, so you need to make those thoughts positive, not negative. If you are one of those individuals who think negative thoughts and comments do not cause any harm, try this experiment (this works better if you are a parent): Make negative comments to your children such as "you can't do that," "you're not good enough," "you always screw that up," or "no wonder you don't have any friends." Hopefully, you don't tell your children those deplorable comments. If you said that to them, can you honestly say that wouldn't have a negative impact on their life? It appears rather logical that if saying negative comments to your children can create negative results, saying negative comments to yourself will create the same effect.

Why do we tend to dwell more on negative things in our lives than on positive? Instead of doing that, try these uplifting tips:

MENTAL BALANCE AND ALIGNMENT

- Whenever something goes wrong, build your positive thoughts by identifying three good things.
- When someone gives you a positive comment, repeat it to yourself during the day.
- Associate with positive people. Charles "Tremendous" Jones states, "In five years, you will be the product of the books you read and the people you associate with." Stay away from anyone who can or will bring you down. There are some people in your life who you have to associate with, but don't take their negative comments and views on life to heart. As the saying goes, "misery loves company."
- Do unto yourself as you do unto others. That is, don't say anything to yourself that you wouldn't say to someone else.

You may think one little negative comment won't affect you. But this one little perceived harmless thought can cause a chain reaction. And like everything, the more you do it, the more it becomes a habit. This is one thing I am guilty of from time to time. Having three little girls is not always conducive to the plans I have set for the day. I may plan to get bills paid, organize my home office, or write a chapter in this book. And if I don't get those things done because of unforeseen obstacles, in the back of my mind (and even in the front), I get a little irritable because I'm thinking about what I want to accomplish. Then I might get in a bad mood or take it out on my kids. But if we realize what we are doing, how that one little event causes a chain reaction in our thinking and action, the bad feelings and thoughts just end right there.

We're beginning to know more than ever about how the mind and body are connected. Our bodies physically change in stressful situations. They will secrete stress hormones, resist insulin uptake, cause inflammation, and decrease immunity. In the short term this is a normal response to survive, but if we are chronically stressed, these changes can cause problems like heart disease, cancer, diabetes, obesity, chronic pain, and a myriad of maladies. If you are constantly bombarding yourself with negative thoughts, are anxious, worried, frustrated, or mad, you increase your chances of contracting diseases.

In our society, it seems that people with a chaotic and stressful life, those who are so busy they don't have time to take care of themselves, are looked up to. They wear this hectic lifestyle like a badge of honor. If you tell them that you're busy, they try to one-up you. That is a lifestyle that should not be revered. Instead of building such a high tolerance to stress, lower it. Don't allow yourself to get to the point where you break down under the pressure of all that is going on around or to you. I see patients every day who have this stress badge and it holds back their health until they learn to manage it.

In the bestselling book and DVD, *The Secret*, it's called the law of attraction, and it's been around for thousands of years. What you think about is what you will attract into your life. If you think you can't be healthy, you won't be. If you tell yourself you have a high stress life, you'll get more stress in your life. You may think you're different, that you can't do it. As Henry Ford said, "Whether you think you can or you think you can't, you're right." I didn't think I could do it; I considered myself a pessimist. But then the more I read and learned and experienced, the more I realized that it is a choice in how you see things. If you want to wallow in your highly stressful, unhealthy, and painful life, you can choose to. But if you want to accept that you can do something to improve your health and life, you can do that too. The first thing is to think and believe you can make it happen, using healthy, positive thoughts because that will lead to positive action. Obstacles will happen in your life that make it harder to be positive, but to create any change or habit, you have to consistently practice.

To help you practice and change the way you talk to yourself, Dr. Wayne Dyer suggests changing self-defeating statements into more powerful, affirming statements in *The Power of Intention*:

I feel uneasy about the state of the economy; I've already lost so much money.
I live in an abundant universe; I choose to think about what I have and I will be fine. The universe will provide.

I have so many things to do that I can never get caught up.

117

I'm at peace in this moment. I'll only think about the thing I'm doing. I will have peaceful thoughts.

I can never get ahead in this job.
I choose to appreciate what I'm doing right now. I'll attract an even greater opportunity.

My health is a huge concern. I worry about getting old and becoming dependent and sick.
I'm healthy, and I think healthy. I live in a universe. I attract healing, and I refuse to anticipate sickness.

My family members are causing me to feel anxious and fearful.
I choose thoughts that make me feel good, and this will help me uplift those family members in need.

I don't deserve to feel good when so many people are suffering.
I didn't come into a world where everyone is going to have the same identical experiences. I'll feel good, and by being uplifted, I'll help eradicate some of the suffering.

I can't be happy when the person I really care about loves another and has abandoned me.
Feeling bad won't change this scenario. I trust that love will return to my life if I'm in harmony with the loving Source. I choose to feel good right now and focus on what I have, rather than what's missing.

The preceding statements could be classified as positive affirmations. I'm not sure if you are familiar with, or remember, the skit on Saturday Night Live with Stuart Smalley called "Daily Affirmations" in which he said, "I'm good enough. I'm smart enough, and doggone it, people like me." When I was a kid watching that, I thought, "This guy's a loser. How could that help?" Now that I have more experience, it makes sense. The thoughts you have in your head will more than likely exhibit themselves in reality. Using positive affirmations will help you get through rough times, to remind yourself that life is good, that you are good, and that you can accomplish your goals.

Noah St. John has an interesting spin on positive affirmations. Usually, positive affirmations are written as statements like, "I am rich", "I am smart", or "I am healthy." But instead of using statements, Mr. St. John puts them in question format, such as "why am I so rich?", "why am I so smart?", or "why am I so healthy?" He calls them positive af*form*ations to help you form those realities. They allow you to think more deeply about why you are those things, and then they can come about even more easily.

Relax...Get to it!

Relaxation is a huge part of de-stressing, and two of my favorite techniques are getting a massage or getting adjusted by a chiropractor. Massage helps you relax, re-align and rejuvenate. There are many positive aspects to receiving massage therapy on an ongoing basis. With the busy lives we lead, we can all benefit from stress management. There are many massage techniques including medical, deep tissue, sports, manual, lymphatic drainage, and prenatal massages. Being a chiropractor, of course I will recommend you get adjusted. The adjustment relieves irritation on your nerves, reduces muscle tension, and improves circulation. For me, the effect of a two-minute adjustment relaxes me more than an hour massage.

Many people wait until they have a few days off or go on vacation to relax. Don't wait that long! Instead of waiting for big blocks of time to relax (which come too infrequently), a much healthier avenue is to take small amounts of time every day to relax. As little as eight minutes a day can change your life. If you don't think you have eight minutes to devote to relaxing and rejuvenating every day because you are too busy, you need to re-assess your priorities. Those eight minutes could turn into hours going to doctors to figure out why you have pain, high blood pressure, or a myriad of other symptoms. Then you will spend way more than eight minutes getting treated for those problems. Take minimal time now and every day so that does not happen.

There are relaxation techniques you can also do by yourself. You may have noticed when you are at work, at home or under mental stress, your shoulders start to creep up toward your ears. Maybe you haven't noticed it, and that's an even bigger problem. The problem is that it happens repeatedly, day after day, and you do not realize it. This stress causes your body to work harder and break down faster. A progressive relaxation technique would be to contract your muscles, starting from your feet and going all the way up to your head. Here is how it works:

- Contract (tighten) the muscles of your toes, feet, and ankles. Hold for five seconds and relax.
- Contract the muscles of your lower legs. Hold for five seconds and relax.
- Contract the muscles of your thighs. Hold for five seconds and relax.
- Contract the muscles of your hips and buttocks. Hold for five seconds and relax.
- Contract the muscles of your low back and stomach. Hold for five seconds and relax.
- Contract the muscles of your chest and shoulder blades. Hold for five seconds and relax.
- Contract the muscles of your shoulders and upper arms. Hold for five seconds and relax.
- Contract the muscles of your forearms and hands. Hold for five seconds and relax.

- Lift your shoulders up toward your ears. Hold for five seconds and relax.
- Contract the muscles of your neck, face, mouth, and head. Hold for five seconds and relax.

This exercise gives your brain and body a comparison of when it is relaxed and when it is not. Your body will better identify those situations when it is not relaxed, and you'll be able to relax your tight muscles. This does not take much time (three to five minutes), but it could be that little thing that changes your life.

Action Steps

1. **Read inspiring books.** One of the best books written for positive thinking is called *The Power of Positive Thinking* from Norman Vincent Peel. It was written in the 1950's, but all of the principles apply today. Two other recommendations are *The Power of Intention* by Dr. Wayne Dyer and *8 Minute Meditation* by Victor Davich. All of these books will clear your mind and give you insight to the power your thoughts have.

2. **Breathe.** It may sound funny, but many people forget how to breathe. They hold their breath and are not even aware of it. In the morning and at night before bed, go outside (as long as it's not too cold) and take five to ten deep breaths. Breathe from the stomach and diaphragm. As

you breathe in, your stomach should protrude. As you breathe out, your stomach should go in. This exercise not only helps your mind, it helps get oxygen to into your body and helps relax and strengthen vital muscles throughout your trunk. Clear your mind at two important parts of your day.

3. **Write it down.** Making lists helps you identify problems and solutions. Do not try to keep it in your head, because doing so distracts your thinking and focus. Also, it causes more mental stress. Once you get it down on paper, you can actually see it in front of you and you can address it without it taking up brain space. These don't just have to be "bad" lists, either. I recommend buying a journal to write these in. Here are a few lists to make:

- Identify the stresses in your life. List the types of physical, chemical, and mental/emotional stresses in your life. You will see how these affect your health on a daily basis. (Many stresses will be discussed in Chapter 8).
- List the three most stressful moments you've had today, and how you reacted to them. It will help you see a pattern and how to address it.
- List seven things that make you really happy and review them regularly. This is your "Happy List."

I hope that you will come up with many more than seven.

- List five things you want to accomplish today and then prioritize them. And, on a Sunday, list at least seven things you accomplished during the week. Do not stress about what you did not accomplish; only feel happy about what you did.

- List your goals. When do you want to accomplish your goals? Why are they important to you? If you know the "why," it will keep you striving toward your goals. Set a goal in the seven different spheres of your life - Personal, Family, Career, Mental/Emotional, Physical, Spiritual, Financial - and I will give examples to help you. Your goals should be SMART - Specific, Measurable, Attainable, Realistic, and Time sensitive. Once you know your goals, you can work backwards to determine which little steps you must take to accomplish them. "The major reason for setting a goal is for what it makes of you to accomplish it. What it makes of you will always be of far greater value than what you get." –Jim Rohn

Personal Goals. These could be places to see, things to do, people to meet. Examples: "My goal is to attend a Final Four weekend by April 15, 2012." "My goal is to go on one vacation per year for at least a week starting in 2008."

Family Goals. What do you want to accomplish as it relates to your family? Examples: "My goal is to spend at least 30 quality minutes a day with my girls." "My goal is to have one date with my wife every month."

Career/Professional Goals. Think about where you want to be in your career, how far you want to go. Examples: "My goal is to be vice president of my company by the end of 2013." "My goal is to start my own company by June 30, 2010." "My goal is to write a book by October 31, 2010."

Mental/Emotional Goals. What things can you do to help expand your mind? Examples: "My goal is to read two books per month in 2010." "My goal is to meditate every day for two months starting May 15, 2010."

Physical Goals. This is the one most people think about with goal setting. Examples: "My goal is to lose two pounds per week over the next two months." "My goal is to increase my vertical jump to 30 inches by December 31, 2009." "My goal is to compete in a triathlon by December 31, 2012."

Spiritual Goals. How can you further your understanding of the non-physical world? Examples: "My goal is to attend mass every

Sunday for two months starting June 1, 2010."
"My goal is to give thanks to God before every
meal starting today." "My goal is to give $1000
per year to charity."

Financial Goals. This is not the same as career
goals. Examples: "My goal is to retire by the age
of 55." "My goal is to buy a beach house in North
Carolina by August 16, 2016." "My goal is to save
$50 dollars per week for the next 12 weeks."

4. **Contact and reconnect with people you've lost
   touch with and would like to talk to or spend
   time with.** Or just spend time with people you
   like being with. When we're alone, we tend to
   get a little more depressed. You may like having
   your alone time, but you still need loved ones in
   your life. I am not talking about the complainers,
   drainers, and others that bring you down. You
   want to have positive relationships because if
   they are negative, that's more detrimental than
   not having any relationships at all. It could be
   family members, friends, neighbors, or
   coworkers that provide encouragement and
   assurance to you.

5. **Do not watch the news or read the newspaper.**
   The news focuses mostly on the negative events
   that happen in the world. If something is bad
   enough, you'll find out about it. Somebody will

tell you about it. You don't have to seek it out by watching the news or reading the newspaper. If you are busy like most people, why waste thirty minutes or more each day reading or watching information and events that will bring you down?

CHILDREN'S HEALTH: WHAT THEY AREN'T TELLING YOU

I THOUGHT LONG AND HARD about writing this piece. I didn't want to sound like a sanctimonious know-it-all. But because of my position, I feel compelled to share the knowledge I've gained through my research and studies. Apparently, as parents and role models, you are not given this information through other avenues. These avenues include, but are not limited to, your doctors, pediatricians, other parents, and even the media.

Believe it or not, drugs and surgery are not the first line of defense for whatever ails your children. It is becoming commonplace to have drugs and surgery prescribed for your children, especially for ear infections. Please understand that if you have done this, I am not blaming or reprimanding you. I hold responsible those who have forced these invasive and potentially dangerous treatments on you, leading you to believe those are the only options. Unfortunately, pediatricians are in the forefront. However, I am not condemning the entire pediatric profession. As a chiropractor, I know what it's like to be indicted for the indiscretions of others in my profession. There are excellent, well-educated, caring pediatricians, just as there are such chiropractors.

Ear Infections

Antibiotics are commonly prescribed for acute otitis media (a.k.a. ear infections), despite evidence of poor outcomes and high complication rates associated with their use. A study by Garbutt et al in *Pediatrics* reported "several authors have advocated restriction of antibiotic treatment for acute otitis media to children . . . under two years of age, although, surprisingly, there is virtually no empirical evidence as to the effectiveness of antibiotic treatment in these children." Results showed only slight differences between the antibiotic (amoxicillin) and placebo groups. At day 11, no significant differences in symptoms and ear examination results were observed in children with ear infections. Amoxicillin use shortened the duration of fever by only one day, but no differences were noted between the two groups in terms of crying or pain. The study also points out that several literature reviews have shown that the effectiveness of antibiotics for acute otitis media is limited. Furthermore, evidence of the effectiveness of antibiotics for this common condition is not conclusive in children under two years of age. Watchful waiting beginning at the first visit is advised.

"A series of controlled studies have revealed that the use of antibiotics for treatment of ear infections makes no difference in terms of the important outcomes -- hearing loss, spread of infection, or mastoiditis. Their use may slightly shorten the duration of pain and infection, but the trade-off is that the antibiotics also reduce the body's natural immune response. Consequently, in order to slightly reduce the duration of the infection, you increase the possibility that the child will have new infections every four to six weeks." This is according to Dr. Robert Mendelsohn, a renowned pediatrician.

One would surely think that surgical intervention with ear tubes is warranted and verified by research, but this is definitely not the case. When both ears are infected and a tube is inserted into only one of them, the outcome of both ears is nearly identical. Interestingly, this procedure is used to cure recurrent otitis media, but one of the side effects is acute otitis media. If your child has recurrent ear infections, it is most likely due to allergies or the antibiotics he or she was previously given. Inserting ear tubes has "replaced tonsillectomy as the favorite of pediatricians, but there is no reliable scientific evidence that it will do any good, and there's considerable evidence that it may cause further harm." Again, this statement is from Dr. Mendelsohn.

Here is more evidence:

"Antibiotic therapy is not an effective treatment against ear infections and rates of recurrent infections are significantly higher in children who have been treated with antibiotics. Prescribing antibiotics for colds, upper respiratory tract infections or bronchitis

does little or nothing to treat the problem. These conditions are caused by viruses and antibiotic drugs have little or no effect on viruses."
—Journal of the American Medical Association, Dec. 18, 1991

"The uncontrolled and inappropriate use of antibiotics is highly responsible for the development of new strains of antibiotic-resistant bacteria. Overuse of antibiotics has been shown to weaken the body's natural immune system."
—World Health Report 1996, World Health Organization

"Prescribing antibiotics immediately increased the number of children who had diarrhea. Immediate prescribing also increased parents' belief in effectiveness in antibiotics and their intention to consult their doctor with the same problem in the future. By prescribing early for a SELF LIMITING ILLNESS, *doctors fuel expectation and probably encourage the cycle of reattendance. This will maintain* PARENTAL DEMAND *for antibiotics, which encourages the* PRESCRIBING OF ANTIBIOTICS AND FURTHER DEVELOPMENT OF ANTIBIOTIC RESISTANCE.*"
—Dr. Little, British Medical Journal, 2001

Common Cold (Upper Respiratory Infections)

Children receive a disproportionate number of prescriptions for antibiotics, particularly to treat upper respiratory infections (URIs). Many of these prescriptions are unnecessary because they are given for viral infections such as the common cold. The Centers for Disease Control and Prevention, the American Academy of Pediatrics, and the American Academy of Family Physicians have all published guidelines to reduce inappropriate antibiotic prescriptions in an attempt to prevent antimicrobial resistance. An astounding 97% of physicians agreed that antibiotic overuse is a major factor contributing to resistance; 83% agreed that the issue of potential resistance should be a consideration when deciding whether to prescribe antibiotics. However, many reported practices and doctors did not adhere to the recently published recommendations for judicious antibiotic use. For example, 86% prescribed antibiotics for bronchitis regardless of the duration of cough and 42% prescribed antibiotics for the common cold. And we already determined this is an unnecessary practice.

Approximately 60 to 75% of URIs in preschool-aged children are caused by viruses. According to a report in the April 1999 issue of *Pediatrics*, "Despite a great deal of evidence that antimicrobials have no role in the treatment of most of these infections, 46% of children and 52% of adults diagnosed with URIs leave the

132

physician's office with an antibiotic prescription." Parental expectations also play a role in the prescription of antibiotics:

- When physicians thought a parent wanted an antibiotic for viral complaints, they prescribed them 62% of the time, compared with only 7% of the time when they did not think the parent wanted antibiotics.
- Physicians were also more likely to give a bacterial diagnosis when they thought parents expected antibiotics (70% vs. 31%).
- Interestingly, actual parental expectations for receiving antibiotics were not associated with physician prescribing patterns.

With increasing bacterial resistance resulting in increased health problems and health care costs, antibiotic over prescribing has become a critical issue worldwide.

Acute Sinusitis

Acute sinusitis, or inflammation of the membranes lining the sinuses, is one of the most prevalent childhood ailments for which antibiotics are routinely prescribed. However, it is unclear whether antibiotics offer significant clinical benefit. Guidelines exist that recommend the use of drugs such as amoxicillin as first-line defense for children who have runny nose and cough without improvement for 10 to 14 days. One study showed that for children diagnosed with acute sinusitis, neither amoxicillin nor amoxicillin-clavulanate (both antibiotics) offered any clinical benefit compared with placebo. Plus, there was no significant difference in improvement rates 14 days after the initiation of treatment.

Behavioral Problems

Attention deficit-hyperactivity disorder (ADHD) is a commonly diagnosed childhood condition. Three- to six-fold increases in the number of patient visits for ADHD and the number of prescriptions for Ritalin have been noted since 1990. Despite the lack of data, experts contend that 3 to 5% of the U.S. pediatric population suffers from ADHD. Recently, the National Institutes of Health recognized that possible over-diagnosis and over treatment of ADHD might be an important public health issue.

A study involving nearly 30,000 grade-school students in two U.S. cities (grades two through five) evaluated the extent of medication use for ADHD. Nurses recorded the number of students who received ADHD medication in school. By fifth grade, 18 to 20% of Caucasian boys were receiving medication. That's one out of every five children! In addition, those students who were "young for one's grade" were also more likely to receive ADHD medication.

Short-term benefits of medication seem to be supported by the literature, but the long-term effects are largely undocumented. Further research on ADHD treatment/therapy approaches is necessary to ensure appropriate use of stimulant medications and non-pharmacologic interventions. All avenues must be explored before embarking on a regimen of potentially harmful drugs, especially in young children. We need to ask ourselves, "Do they have ADHD, or are they just being kids?" More often than not, it is the latter.

Here are more startling revelations about prescription drug use in America's youth:

- 60% of children in the Texas foster care system are being drugged with powerful psychotropic drugs, most of which have not been tested in or approved for use in_children. Two powerful antipsychotic drugs -- Risperdal and Zyprexa -- made up half of the drugs prescribed to foster children in Texas. These two drugs have been approved only for adults for the treatment of psychosis (primarily schizophrenia), yet children as young as four were receiving these powerful, mind-altering drugs.
- Between 2000 and 2003, the use of psychotropic drugs among teenagers increased three-fold, and the number of children treated for "severe behavioral conditions" related to conduct disorder and autism jumped more than 60%.
- The FDA estimates 11 million antidepressant prescriptions were written in 2003 for under 19 year olds -- a 27% increase in 3 years.

- Drugs used primarily to treat ADHD increased the most. In 5- to 9-year-old children, the use of drugs increased 85%, and in preschoolers, usage was up 49%.

- Physicians prescribe mind-altering drugs even as they know that the developing brain is undergoing extraordinary changes. They acknowledge: "we have very little information about the long-term impact of treatment with these drugs early in development."

- Even infants and toddlers are prescribed Prozac with the blessing of the medical / psychiatric establishment. In 1998, an FDA contracted survey found that 3,000 Prozac prescriptions had been written for infants! In March 2004, the US FDA issued extensive bold warnings about the increased risk of suicidal behavior in both children and adults who take an antidepressant. In October 2004, the FDA issued black box warnings about the two-fold increased risk of suicidal behavior in youth taking any antidepressant, including Prozac.

- Antipsychotics are the most powerful, most toxic psychotropic drugs that have neither been tested in, nor approved for use in children, yet they are the second most widely prescribed drugs for children. Antipsychotics are the fourth highest selling class of prescribed drugs in the US; sales in 2002 reached $6.4 billion.

Youth Exercise Guidelines

Over the years, it's been common knowledge among parents and others that children should not lift weights. Some of the fears are that it will stunt their growth, damage their growth plates, and it is unsafe and dangerous. However, recent research is dispelling these misconceptions. Evidence is demonstrating that lifting weights, or strength training, increases bone strength along with having many other benefits.

Strength training is a method of training designed to increase an individual's ability to resist and exert force. It encompasses using anything that provides resistance, such as your own body weight, dumbbells, barbells, medicine balls, elastic bands, machines, etc. Now let's put this in terms of children. Think about how many times a day children engage in weight lifting (or strength training) activities. They squat, lunge, pull, and push all the time. These all involve lifting weight, the children's own weight, but that isn't thought of as dangerous. From the moment babies can crawl, then learn how to walk, they are lifting weights. In essence, they are strength training.

Strength training gets confused with weight lifting and bodybuilding, which are specific sports. When parents hear "lifting weights", they think of big power lifters or bodybuilders lifting tremendous amounts of weight over their head. Television and magazines show competitive power lifters straining to lift enormous amounts of weight or bodybuilders posing with their muscles bulging. It's no wonder they've developed negative attitudes toward children and strength training. Many coaches and parents think that is what strength training is, but there's much more to it than that. The goal of strength training does not have to be lifting maximum amounts of weight or building huge muscles. We should not confuse strength training with maximal-type exercises performed during competitive weightlifting or power lifting competitions.

Some benefits of strength training in youths are:

- *Increased musculoskeletal system function.* The musculoskeletal system consists of the muscles, tendons, ligaments, and bones. Proper strength training programs increase muscle strength, muscle endurance, and bone strength. This is contrary to the belief that strength training stunts growth or reduces bone formation. Increased function of muscles, tendons, and bones also means that joint stability is increased.

- *Prevention of overuse injuries.* Most overuse injuries occur to the musculoskeletal system. So if your musculoskeletal function improves, obviously the chance of injury lessens. According to the American College of Sports Medicine, children could prevent about 50% of overuse injuries in youth sports if they emphasized general fitness over sport specific skills.

- *Improved performance.* If the muscles are working optimally and injury risk is low, your performance in life and sports will improve. You will be able to practice and play longer, and your muscles will respond more readily.

- *Positive attitude*. Childhood is the essential time to develop lifelong attitudes and active behaviors. Therefore, this is a great time to introduce strength training. It provides sedentary students with positive after school activities in contrast to video games and watching television. They enjoy the purposeful exercise, experience personal improvement, and train with friends in a supportive environment. This improves self–esteem, especially in overweight youths. This population is usually not as adept at the endurance activities, but they shine in strength training because they are stronger. It improves their body composition by increasing their metabolism and burning excess calories.

The safety of strength training is the paramount issue with parents and coaches. The biggest concern is damage to the growth cartilage. A few cases have reported growth plate fractures in children who lifted weights, but most of these occurred due to improper training technique, excessive weight used, and lack of qualified supervision. To provide a safe training program, it's important to follow the youth strength training guidelines set out by various health and fitness organizations such as: National Strength and Conditioning Association, the American Orthopedic Society for Sports Medicine, American Academy of Pediatrics, Society of Pediatric Orthopeadics, American

College of Sports Medicine, President's Council on Physical Fitness and Sports, U.S. Olympic Committee, and National Athletic Trainers Association. Close supervision of children during their strength training sessions and ensuring they follow a structured program will minimize the risk of injury.

Remember that children are not miniature adults and therefore should not follow standard adult workout programs. Before children engage in any strength training program, it's important they are ready for it. Ask these questions to determine if children will benefit from a strength training program (taken from *Strength Training for Young Athletes*):

- Is the child mentally and physically ready to participate?
- What are the goals of the child?
- Which program should the child follow?
- Do the child and supervisor understand proper lifting techniques and safety spotting techniques for each exercise?
- Does the child understand safety considerations for every exercise?
- Does the child have a balanced physical exercise training program including cardiovascular activities and flexibility exercises?

Strength Training Guidelines

Many times coaches and parents don't know where to begin. These guidelines provide a basic outline on appropriate techniques to use. First, children need to learn how to lift their own bodyweight. If they cannot use correct form, then they should not use an external load like barbells or dumbbells, because it will accentuate the improper form and increase the risk of injury. Research has shown that musculoskeletal injury rarely occurs, but a majority of the cases where injury occurred are linked with maximal overhead lifts. Of course, most injuries occur as a result of poor supervision of the children. Too many children, as well as coaches, get caught up in the amount of weight they can lift even at the start of a program. They have to realize that if they develop perfect form first, they will be able to lift more weight later.

Here are some guidelines that parents and coaches should follow when incorporating a youth strength training program:

- Pre-pubescent children will gain strength by improving the ability of the nervous system, not by increasing the size of the muscle. Muscles don't really grow until puberty, when testosterone, estrogen, and progesterone increase. Thus, they do not need to lift heavy weights.
- Design a program based on each child's individual needs that involves proper exercise technique.

141

- Proper progression, program monitoring, and supervision are essential to the needs of the children.
- Children should lift weights that they can lift 8 to 15 times. The age when a child can start lifting heavier weights depends on individual maturation and training experience.
- Increase repetitions before increasing weight. Increase the weight gradually as strength improves. Increasing from 20 pounds to 30 pounds is a 50% increase in weight, which is a large jump in weight. Increase the weight by 5 to 10%.
- Two to three training sessions per week is adequate.
- Children should have a thorough exam prior to starting an exercise program.
- Do not compare one child to another. Each child progresses and grows at a different rate.

Proper progression and patience are key. Just as you wouldn't expect a young student to pass a grade in six weeks, you shouldn't expect them to attain perfect fitness in six weeks. To become good at anything takes time and effort over several years. A younger, inexperienced child does not need to do sophisticated, complex exercises to make progress. For example, many youths perform power cleans (at the instruction of either coaches or teachers) before knowing how to correctly perform a squat or deadlift, which are preliminary exercises to the power clean. Trying to perform complex exercises at this stage often leads to injury or gives little benefit because technique is too poor to improve.

Strength training is a safe and effective activity for children to participate in. As long as the guidelines are followed, children should enjoy and flourish in a well-designed strength training program. It is important to remember that health and fitness is not a short-term investment. Do not expect to achieve perfection in months; it takes years of smart and hard work. Therefore, introducing strength training to children helps them develop active behaviors that will last a lifetime.

Machines Are Not As Safe

Have you seen Rocky IV? It was the one with the Russian, Ivan Drago. In his training, Rocky went old-school, running in the snow, chopping wood, chopping down trees, lifting and towing rocks, pulling a sled in the snow, climbing snowy mountains. Drago was in the comfortable confines of a state-of-the-art training complex, running indoors, running on a treadmill, using weight-training machines. Guess who won? I know, I know; it's a movie. I completely understand that point, but I feel in this case, art imitates life. Believe me, I don't want to oversimplify athletic training, but Rocky's and Drago's respective training regimens are a great example of how free weight, non machine-based training is more beneficial, especially with children.

A free weight, non machine-based training program relies mainly on body weight, dumbbells, barbells, medicine balls, elastic bands, and cables as its primary sources of resistance. These tools are more efficient than machines for a few reasons. First, you have to stabilize

143

yourself while using free weights, instead of the machine providing the stability and guiding the motion (which does not happen in life or sport). This is important in injury prevention, which we will discuss below. Second, the abilities you gain with free weights transfer more readily onto the playing field. Third, free weight training allows you to work unilaterally (that is one side of the body at a time) much more easily than with machines. Obviously, this is important because when one side creates force, the other side stabilizes, as in kicking, throwing, and swinging. Last, free weights can also work in the transverse plane (rotational movements), but it's very difficult for machines to produce the same action. Over 85% of the core musculature is oriented horizontally or diagonally, so we are designed to rotate. Therefore, you need to train in this plane of motion.

Most importantly, a free weight-based program prevents injuries, especially overuse injuries. Overuse injuries are on the rise in young athletes. Recent research indicates 30 to 50% of all pediatric sports injuries are due to overuse. So what are overuse injuries? Overuse injuries occur when a tissue (muscle, ligament, or tendon) is injured due to repetitive sub-maximal loading. In other words, performing an action over and over and over and over causes excessive wear and tear. This repetitive activity will fatigue a tissue. With sufficient recovery, the tissue can get stronger and undergo further activity without injury. However, without adequate recovery, microtrauma and inflammation develop, causing damage to the local tissue. Continued repetitive activity causes clinical injury and recurrent problems leading to weakness, loss of flexibility, and chronic pain. Therefore, *chronic* degeneration is the primary problem in overuse injuries, not necessarily the *acute* tissue inflammation.

Several factors contribute to overuse. These are summarized in the table below.

Intrinsic Factors	Extrinsic Factors
Growth (susceptibility of growth cartilage to repetitive stress, inflexibility, muscle imbalance)	Too rapid training progression
	Inadequate rest
Prior injury	Inappropriate equipment
Inadequate conditioning	Incorrect sport technique
Anatomic malalignment	Uneven or hard surfaces
Menstrual dysfunction	Adult or peer pressure
Psychological factors	

According to the American College of Sports Medicine, children could prevent about 50% of overuse injuries in youth sports if they emphasized general fitness over sport specific skills. Children will benefit from a general strength and endurance program before beginning a rigorous specific training program. However, unfit children may lack the proprioceptive skills (body awareness) and have too weak or inflexible musculoskeletal tissues to withstand these loading forces. Therefore, gradual training progression with adequate recovery periods will help prevent overuse injuries. Be aware that training programs for adults are not appropriate for young athletes because of their varied physical and emotional maturity. At this stage (6 to 13 years of age), sport specialization should also be discouraged.

This brings us back to the free weight versus machine training debate. As mentioned, part of the training program includes general strength development. You could use machines, but why would you want to. True, machines do build strength, but in addition to the aforementioned limitations, they don't increase balance, flexibility, or stability. And these are integral in preventing overuse injuries. Remember, machines provide the stability and guide the motion for you. Problems may arise with excessive machine use because many of the overuse injuries occur in the stabilizer muscles like the rotator cuff, knee stabilizers, hip stabilizers, and deep low back muscles. Machines do *not* train these muscles very well.

Just because something has been done a certain way for years and years does not mean it's the right or best way to do it. If that's the way it's supposed to be, we would never have any change, we wouldn't try to make anything better. Baseball players wouldn't wear helmets, football helmets wouldn't have facemasks, basketball players would still wear Converse All Stars, doctors would still use leeches, athletes would still take salt tablets to prevent dehydration, and youths wouldn't strength train.

Approximately 35 million children and young adults between 6 and 21 years of age participate in sports, including six to eight million in school programs. If we do not start teaching youths correct training principles, they may sustain injuries that will affect them the rest of their lives. So please look beyond what you have been told in the past and think logically before engaging your children in a machine-based training program.

Action Steps

1. Get a specific biomechanical, structural, and neurological exam to determine if there are any structural imbalances present in your child. Chiropractors or some physical therapists conduct these exams most thoroughly.

Physical imbalances can happen from birth. This is called Traumatic Birth Syndrome (TBS) and occurs when:

- Drugs are used during labor.
- An epidural is used.
- Labor is induced.
- The baby is in a difficult position during pregnancy and delivery.
- Labor is long and difficult.
- Vacuum extraction, forceps or a C-section is used for delivery.

A Cesarean (C-section) delivery is no less traumatic. The baby does not magically appear when the doctor makes the incision. The doctor still has to pull on the baby's head and neck, which can cause an imbalance. In addition, a C-section is not as healthy for the baby. There is a reason the baby is supposed to have a normal vaginal birth.

Even so-called "normal" birth can cause spinal injuries from the force of contractions against the child's head, neck, and spine. These spinal injuries caused from the birth process may go undetected and show no signs or symptoms for years. They do, however, cause interference with function and healing, causing many health problems including colic, ear infections, asthma, allergies, constant colds, hyperactivity, and poor health and vitality in general. Left uncorrected, Traumatic Birth Syndrome can lead to premature spinal aging and postural problems and can affect your child's future health.

Dr. Abraham Towbin from the Harvard School of Medicine stated, "research indicates that the major cause of spinal subluxation [imbalance] in infants is childbirth. Stressing the need for correction from birth so that irreversible subluxation degeneration changes do not occur. Nerve system injury through cervical spine trauma at birth causes abnormal function, abnormal behavior, and early death (SIDS)."

When is it easier to get rid of a problem? After a day of having it, or after 20 years of having it? And that's a big problem, because many children walk around with these structural imbalances that build up over a lifetime, and their bodies wear down a lot quicker. So that's why it's important to get a structural exam to see if there are any imbalances present.

2. **Get moderate regular exercise.** This is the same as for adults, but children are not mini-adults. Exercise programs for adults should not be used for children. Refer back to the Young Exercise Guidelines section of this chapter. This applies to all children. You have to make exercise fun. Children have many more choices today than in the past. There are computers, the internet, video games, and cell phones, which all take away play time. We used to play active games, usually outside. Games like freeze tag, red light green light, dodgeball, jump rope, and making obstacle courses are all fun and easy to play. Create family activities such as going for walks or bike rides after dinner instead of sitting in front of the TV.

A common mistake is making exercise "not fun," and even worse, a punishment. This is more prevalent in the athletic world. I remember when I played sports, if we made a mistake or lost a game, we would have to run. That creates a program in children's minds that exercise is bad. "If I lose I have to exercise." This still occurs every day in youth practices. Instead of using exercise as punishment, use exercise as a reward. For example, the winning team *gets* to play a game like tag or lightning or another game that they like. The key is to make it fun and active. The more creative the better!

3. **Eat nutritious foods.** You must set a great example for your kids, especially when it comes to food. You are the adult. It is your job to keep them safe and be the bad guy or gal sometimes. Our society is loaded with processed foods that are marketed toward kids, and it is very hard to say "no" repeatedly. The colorful boxes with their favorite cartoon or TV character have no nutritional food in them. They are all highly processed and stripped of their nutrients, regardless of what it says on the box. Stick with the raw fruits and vegetables, organic produce and dairy, and nuts and seeds. Consult the Nutrition chapter for more fresh ideas. It is even more important for your children to eat nutritious foods than for you.

4. **Give them positive reinforcement every day.** You want them to live in a healthy environment. If you keep putting them down, telling them they can't do things, they're going to believe you. "Sticks and stones will break my bones, but words will never hurt me." How wrong are those words? Whether you believe it or not, your children look up to you. Make a point to tell and show your kids that you love them, and that they're safe, because that's the most important

thing. You may think they know it, but it's something you need to tell them throughout their lives. Make sure they know it, and believe it!

"The Doctor of the future will give no medicine but will interest his patients in the care of the human frame, in diet, and in the cause and prevention of disease."

—Thomas Edison

STRESSOR LIST

"I DON'T KNOW WHAT I did to make it hurt." That's a statement I hear almost every day. The following list consists of various physical, chemical, and emotional/mental stresses you potentially put onto your body, currently or in the past. Repeated abuse of these stressors causes your body to get out of balance, making it more susceptible to symptoms and disease.

To give you an idea of how these affect your health, imagine your body as an empty glass underneath a leaky faucet. Every drop that goes in the glass is a stressor you are putting on or in your body. Some drops are bigger than others. Not until the water overflows will you get any symptoms or diseases. The goal is to fix the leak and dump the water out of the glass by doing healthy activities that, of course, are the opposite of these stressors.

Go through this list and make note of all of the ones you are guilty of. The more you check off, the unhealthier you will be.

Physical

- Not exercising at a moderate intensity for 20-30 minutes three to five times per week. (Moderate intensity means "slightly out of breath" to "can't hold conversation": running, walking briskly, jogging, strength/circuit training, swimming, yoga, Pilates, biking, skiing, aerobics, elliptical, treadmill, Stairmaster, exercise videos/DVDs).
- Not performing stretching or flexibility exercises, including massage or chiropractic adjustments.
- Not getting at least six hours of sleep at night.
- Not taking naps.
- Performing repetitive movements like painting, gardening, shoveling, landscaping, throwing, overhead activities.
- Sitting down most of the day, especially at a computer.
- Talking with the phone between your shoulder and ear.
- Sitting on a wallet.
- Standing in one position most of the day.
- Using improper bending techniques *repetitively* or when lifting something heavy.
- Holding or carrying objects repetitively, like children, boxes, equipment, laundry, groceries, or luggage
- Having trouble falling asleep.
- Sleeping on your stomach.
- Sleeping in an unsupportive bed, couch, or chair.
- Having poor posture including:

Head out in front of your shoulders

One shoulder higher than the other

Shoulders rolled forward

   Flat feet

   Knees rotated inward or outward (knock-knees or bow legs)

   One leg shorter than the other

- Past serious medical ailments, accidents, or injuries (heart attack, cancer, car accident, or injury requiring surgery, etc).
- Being pregnant.
- Delivery process for mom and baby.
- Falling down, especially when learning to walk.
- Carrying a backpack.
- Wearing unsupportive shoes, especially while exercising, walking, or standing.
- Wearing high heels.
- Not wearing foot orthotics to support your foot arches.
- Having an eating disorder.
- Being overweight or obese.
- Sports injuries.
- Performing *repetitive* movements required in sports including:

❖ Archery	❖ Football (Gridiron)	❖ Sailing
❖ Australian Rules Football	❖ Golf	❖ Shooting
	❖ Gymnastics	❖ Soccer
❖ Badminton	❖ Handball	❖ Softball
		❖ Surfing

- ❖ Baseball
- ❖ Basketball
- ❖ Bowling
- ❖ Boxing
- ❖ Canoe/Kayak
- ❖ Cricket
- ❖ Cycling
- ❖ Disc Sports
- ❖ Diving
- ❖ Equestrian
- ❖ Fencing
- ❖ Hockey
- ❖ Horse Racing
- ❖ Ice Hockey
- ❖ Lawn Bowling
- ❖ Martial Arts
- ❖ Motorsports – Motorcycling, Drag racing, Freestyle Motocross
- ❖ Rowing
- ❖ Rugby League
- ❖ Swimming
- ❖ Table Tennis
- ❖ Tennis
- ❖ Triathlon
- ❖ Volleyball
- ❖ Water polo
- ❖ Weightlifting
- ❖ Winter Sports
- ❖ Wresting

- ❖ Adventure Sports
- Backpacking
- Bodyboarding
- Bungee Jumping
- Canyoning
- Caving/Spelunking, Cave diving
- Cycling - Mountain Biking, BMX freestyle
- Dog sledding
- Extreme skiing
- Four Wheel Driving
- Free-diving
- Gliding
- Hang gliding
- Hiking, Hill Walking, Trekking
- Horseback Riding
- Hunting
- Kneeboarding
- Mountaineering / Mountain Climbing
- Paintball
- Parachuting / skydiving
- Parasailing, Paragliding
- Rafting
- Rappelling
- Rock-climbing
- Roller derby
- Sailing and Windsurfing
- Scuba Diving and Snorkeling
- Skateboarding
- Skiboarding
- Skiing, Barefoot skiing
- Slamball
- Snow shoeing
- Snowboarding
- Snowmobiling
- Street luge
- Surfing
- Unicycling
- Wakeboarding
- Water skiing
- White water rafting
- Whitewater kayaking

Chemical

- Not eating raw, fresh fruits every day.
- Not eating raw, fresh vegetables every day.
- Not eating leafy vegetables regularly.
- Not eating almonds, walnuts, flaxseeds regularly.
- Not drinking any milk.
- Not eating fresh fish.
- Not eating fresh, organic, skinless chicken or turkey multiple times per week.
- Not eating cage free, organic Omega-3 eggs.
- Not eating extra virgin olive oil, high oleic expeller pressed safflower or sunflower oil, especially with cooking
- Not drinking enough water every day.
- Not taking any supplements or vitamins daily.
- Not eating breakfast.
- Not eating any fats.
- Drinking non-organic milk, cheese, sour cream, yogurt, and other dairy products.
- Eating too much soy and soy products.
- Eating and drinking diet, light, and no fat products.
- Eating sugar coated cereals.
- Eating junk food like potato chips, cookies, crackers, doughnuts, cake, ice cream, desserts, candy, candy bars, syrups.
- Eating "white" processed foods (enriched white bread, pasta noodles, rice, bagels, muffins, pancakes, waffles)

- Eating whole grains such as whole wheat flour, oat bran, whole wheat pasta, whole wheat bread excessively or never.
- Eating ground red meat like hamburgers multiple times per week.
- Eating non-organic lean red meat multiple times per week.
- Eating organic red meat multiple times per week or never.
- Eating processed meat such as bacon, sausage, pork, lunch meat/turkey, hot dogs.
- Eating condiments such as ketchup, mustard, creamy salad dressings, or mayonnaise excessively.
- Eating butter or margarine.
- Eating fried foods.
- Eating "fast food."
- Drinking soda, especially diet sodas.
- Drinking alcohol.
- Drinking caffeine.
- Drinking energy drinks.
- Using artificial sweeteners like Equal, Splenda.
- Salting your foods excessively.
- Taking prescription medication, over-the-counter drugs (Tylenol, ibuprofen, aspirin, etc), or illegal drugs (marijuana, cocaine, heroine, etc.)
- Using tobacco such as chew, dip, cigarettes, or cigars.
- Skipping meals.

- Being exposed to industrial or agricultural chemicals like solvents, cleaning fluids, paint fumes, plant sprays, pesticides, or fertilizers.
- Being a lifetime dieter.

Mental/Emotional
- Not making time for rest and relaxation.
- Not using appropriate methods to relieve stress or manage stress like deep breathing, meditation, massage, or positive thinking.
- Not regularly seeing close friends and family members with whom you have good relationships.
- Not being involved in activities in which you help others.
- Not liking your job or career.
- Not thinking positively; expecting the worst.
- Having a high amount of stress in your life such as finances, job, getting along with people, family, being happy with yourself, the future.
- Being cynical and disenchanted.
- Being irritable and short-tempered.
- Being mentally sluggish or having poor concentration.
- Having a decreased sex drive.
- Having poor health (yours or your family's).
- Procrastinating.
- Bottling up emotions and allowing events to build up in your mind.
- Associating with negative people.

- Having unsupportive home or work life (spouse, employer, children).
- Worrying about your children.
- Feeling overwhelmed because you are so busy.

Consequences of Stressing Your Body:
- Diarrhea
- Constipation
- Bloating/gas
- Dry skin
- Heartburn/reflux
- Light-headed/dizzy
- Colds/flu
- Water retention
- Sinus problems
- Headaches and migraines
- Allergies
- Mood swings
- Muscle twitches
- Irregular periods (females only)
- Bleeding gums
- Shortness of breath
- Easy bruising
- Canker sores
- Brittle nails
- Tingling in fingers/toes
- PMS
- Low immune system (frequent illnesses)
- Nausea
- Cracks on corners of lips

- Diabetes
- Heart disease
- Arthritis or Degenerative Disc Disease
- Joint pain to the fingers, hands, wrists, elbows, shoulders, neck, mid back, low back, ribs, hips, pelvis, knees, ankles, feet, toes
- Osteoporosis
- Hypoglycemia
- High blood pressure
- Stroke
- Eating disorder
- Heart attack
- Cancer
- Sleep apnea
- Thyroid disorder

FREQUENTLY ASKED QUESTIONS

Q: *Why do I have pain? I didn't do anything. I haven't done anything different. I've never had that before.*

A: Let's tackle this one at a time. The reason you have pain is because of the <u>physical</u>, <u>chemical</u>, and <u>emotional</u> stresses that are on your body. Let's start with the physical stress. Physical stress could be any accidents that you've been in, not just recently but honestly, ever. It could be poor posture, sitting at a computer all day, standing on a hard surface, bending all day, how you sleep, yard work, playing sports, golfing, bowling -- the postures and positions that you're in. Chemical stress comes from your diet and what you eat or don't eat, from the drugs -- I mean medications you take. All drugs, whether they're recreational, over-the-counter, or prescription, have side effects. If you're eating too many processed foods or too much sugar, if you smoke, drink a lot of alcohol or soda and not enough water, those are all things that put a chemical stress on your body. Emotional stress is another big factor. That's the stress people are usually referring to when they say, "I'm stressed out." So if you get "stressed out", like frustrated, worried, or mad, whether it be at work, home, or in your car, guess what, that's a stress you're putting on your body. That stress is not good for it and makes it harder for your body to heal. Usually, it is a combination of the physical, chemical, and emotional stresses that determines how we feel and heal, not just one of them.

OK, now you know about these stresses. These stresses cause your body to get imbalanced, especially in your spine, but it could be your knee, shoulder, hip, or any joint, really. When you get these imbalances in your spine, they irritate the nervous system and put pressure on your muscles, ligaments, tendons, and bones. So this stress on these structures, usually over time, will cause poor health and, in turn, pain. So the question is, do you want to correct the actual problem and improve your health so your symptoms go away, or do you just want to treat the symptom, where it will have a much better chance of coming back? If you improve your health, your symptoms will go away. That's what chiropractic is about; improving your health. That works because your nervous system controls your health, how well you heal. It's something we're all born with. If you cut your arm or hand, what happens? It heals; right? Without you having to take anything. Well, that ability comes from the nervous system. Therefore, if your nerves are irritated and your body can't heal itself as well, you won't be healthy. And you'll get symptoms, whether it's pain, headaches, muscle tension, reflux, ear infections, asthma, you name the ailment. So what we do as chiropractors is adjust the spine and take the pressure off the nervous system so your body can heal, get healthy, and your symptoms will go away. We also advise you on exercise and nutrition, because we all know how huge that is in getting and staying healthy. I know that's a long answer for "why do I have pain," but it's very important to understand pain, health, and how even if you don't have pain, that doesn't necessarily mean you're healthy. Just like if you paid off all your debt, it doesn't mean that you are now wealthy. You could be feeling fine one day, and the next day have a heart attack. Did you do something in those 24 hours to cause that heart attack? No. It's something that's been building up over time. Focus on your health and your symptoms go away.

To address the points of you "not doing anything different" or "not doing anything to cause the pain," hopefully, what we just talked about answered that. But if not, let's use a few examples. Most of us have had a cavity in a tooth. What causes the cavity? Is it because you ate something different before the dentist found it? Usually that's not the case; right? It's been happening over time by doing the same

163

thing over and over again. Doing things that are stressful repeatedly is just as bad as doing something different, maybe even worse, because it's harder to identify the problem. It just takes longer and you wonder why you have it. It's the same thing with the rest of your body; if you put stress on your spine and nervous system over and over again, it can and usually does cause a problem. Just because you've never had a certain pain before, like low back pain, headaches, whatever it is, doesn't mean it won't happen. We hear that a lot. "I've never had that before." Well you haven't had the symptom yet, but the problem has been building over time. It's the straw that broke the camel's back, you might say.

Most people haven't had a heart attack before they actually have one. Most problems don't happen overnight. It takes time for those physical, chemical, and emotional stresses to add up and cause symptoms. So the <u>problem</u> is actually there awhile before you actually feel the <u>symptom</u>. That's why how you are feeling does not determine how healthy you are. I know people that are 100 pounds overweight and they say that they feel fine. Does that mean they're healthy? No! They take blood pressure medication, have high cholesterol, diabetes, asthma, etc. But what would happen if they improved their health? If you've ever watched the Biggest Loser, you know what I'm talking about. You see overweight and obese people trying to lose weight and get healthy. I remember one episode where the wife of one of the contestants came to visit after the contestant had lost a lot of weight. She asked him how his asthma was. He said it was gone. How's your reflux? Gone. How's your cholesterol? Normal. And this isn't the exception. That's what happens when you take control of your health and choose to get healthy. It's your choice. It's not anyone else's. If you don't choose to get healthy, whose fault is it? It's not your doctor's, family's, or co-worker's fault. It's yours. We want to empower you to improve your health, not just get rid of pain. If you improve your health, your symptoms go away. That's what we do.

One last thing; sometimes pain is not a bad thing. It's what made you seek care. We'd much rather see you before you're in pain, to see if there is something that needs to be fixed so it has less potential to cause pain, but that's in an ideal world. What if you couldn't feel pain? You probably wouldn't be alive. It's the body's alarm system that something is wrong. So it's important to take care of yourself, even if you don't have any symptoms. It's definitely better to fix or, better yet, prevent a problem so it doesn't become painful. Again, using a weight loss example, do you have to wait until you're 20, 30, or 50 pounds overweight before you exercise? Absolutely not! Hopefully you understand that, and you are equipped with the knowledge of what it takes not just to be pain free, but to be healthy.

Q: *How long will it take for me to get out of pain and get this problem fixed?*

A: A lot of that depends on how long the problem has been there. If it's been there a long enough time to create changes to your spine, you can expect it could take 4 to 12 months for it actually to get fixed. The way we know how long it's been there is through the exam, looking at your posture, taking you through orthopedic and neurological tests, and especially on x-rays. I do want to mention that you typically start <u>feeling</u> better before 4 to 12 months. But feeling better doesn't actually mean the problem is gone, remember. Usually you start feeling better in the first month of care, but that varies from person to person. It takes ligaments 6 to12 months to heal, so that's why it takes awhile for it to get fixed. Now, if there is so much damage and your spine has been out of place for so long that it causes arthritis with bone spurs and disc degeneration, then that may not be able to be corrected. But there are things that you and we can do to manage it so it doesn't degenerate so quickly. So we treat patients with arthritis all the to help take the stress off their body, which caused the arthritis in the first place. The key is to not let it get so bad that it can't be corrected.

Q: *These symptoms are normal because I'm getting old, right?*

A: If that were the case, wouldn't everyone who was the same age have the same problems? I know 70 year olds that are still golfing and exercising without pain. And I know 30 year olds that already have arthritis. Plus, all of your body is the same age, right? Why doesn't everything break down at the same time? It's all because of the stress that is placed on your body. The longer you live with this stress, the faster things will break down. I encourage you not to use that as an excuse. If you do your best to take the stress off your body, your body will not break down as fast. So how do you do that?

Being a chiropractor, of course I'm going to say you need to get adjusted, because that keeps the stress off your nervous system and allows your body to heal itself better. But it's also exercising regularly, the key word being regularly. I know things happen. You go on vacation, get married, or have high stress at work to where you might not be able to workout for a few weeks or months. Does that mean you can never start again? No! I think sometimes people might be afraid of that. I hear them say, "I have a vacation in a month, so I'll start after that." Heck, start now and pick it up when you get back.

Taking stress off your body, namely the chemical stress, also entails having good eating habits. I'm a big "in moderation" guy. Do it in moderation. Eat out once in awhile. Have a hamburger once in awhile. Eat ice cream once a month, whatever it is, but do it in moderation. If you're eating poorly twice a day, eating fast food even once a day, that's not good. Don't try to fix everything all at once with what you're eating. Substitute things here and there to help you create good eating habits. For example, if you drink 3 or 4 sodas a day, substitute water for one of those drinks. Instead of ground beef, try ground chicken. That's a much better way to make it easier for you to stick to it.

It's not about getting old, it's about the stress on your body that causes you to feel bad. Doing things that counteract this stress, like getting chiropractic care, exercising regularly, having good eating habits, and practicing positive thinking will help with how you feel and heal.

Q: *Why do I have to come in 3 times a week? My other chiropractor only adjusted me once a month or whenever I "needed" it for maintenance care after the first few weeks. I feel fine, so why do I need to get adjusted?*

A: Well, what was the goal of that chiropractor? Was it just to get you out of pain, or adjust you until your symptoms went away, and then adjust you once a month or when you felt you "needed" it? I'm a chiropractor and I don't know when I "need" to be adjusted. I can't detect when my body isn't balanced. It also depends on the phase of care that you're in and the type of care you want. If you just want care for your pain, but not to correct the problem, then you usually start off at 3 times per week and then quit once you feel better. If you want corrective care where you're actually fixing the problem and you make the commitment to fix the problem and get healthy, that's when it's 3 times a week for a certain measure of time. Then your frequency of visits cuts back to maybe twice a week, then once a week as your body and spine get more stable.

If we use the weight loss example again, let's say you have a goal to lose 50 pounds. You start exercising and eating better and you lose 10 pounds. You think that's pretty good, so then you slip on the exercising and eating habits and you stay at that weight. That would be similar to the pain relief type of care. Now let's say you keep going and lose the 50 pounds and keep doing what worked, exercising and eating well. That would be like the corrective care type program. You took the steps necessary to reach your goal, you reached it, and now you're going to continue to do what worked. You know that if you slip back into old habits, your weight will come back. That's the same with your health and chiropractic. Your health is your choice. You can

169

choose to do or not to do anything, but there are always consequences to those choices.

I'm sure you've heard that if you go to a chiropractor, you have to go all the time for the rest of your life. Well you don't *have* to. You don't *have* to do anything. Again, if it works and you get healthy, and then you stop, what has a good chance of happening? I'm not saying you have to come in 3 times a week for the rest of your life. But I believe you do need regular checkups to make sure your body is staying balanced. For some it's every week. For others it's every 2 or 3 weeks. It just depends on your body and health, and the stresses that are placed on it. Bottom line is this: I am responsible for teaching you about health and how to get healthy, and showing you the things that will add value to your life. But you are the only one who can take responsibility to change your own health and life.

Q: Do you work on kids? Is it safe?

A: Yes, we treat kids every day – newborns, toddlers, infants, teenagers, you name it. It is a very safe way to help kids get and stay healthy. Many wonder how that works. Heck, even pediatricians question it. I'm going to try and appeal to your logic. The first argument made is that it isn't safe. I guess they think we're going to tear your children's heads off. Remember back when your child was born and how traumatic that was for you and your baby. How much force did they use the get the baby out? The doctor grabs your baby's head and twists, turns, and pulls, then the shoulder gets pushed way down, all to try and get the baby out. I have three girls and I watched them all being delivered. On our first one, they had to use one of those suction cup things to help pull her out because the cord was wrapped around her. So they put that on her head and suctioned to get a good grip on her head and then pulled her out. Our next one was a classic delivery, just like I described, with the doctor pulling on her head with a lot of force. The doctor even put her foot up on the table so she could get more leverage. Our last one was not as extreme, but there it was again with pulling on her head and neck to get her out. If you think C-sections are less traumatic, you are wrong. It's not like they make an incision and poof the baby just pops out. Do you think with all of that trauma that something could get out of whack in your kid's spine? Heck yeah!

Now let's take this back to chiropractic. We don't put anywhere near the force that children get when they're delivered. We use gentle, non-aggressive techniques on their spines. My kids have been getting adjusted since they were three days old. You need to ask yourself, would we adjust our own kids if it wasn't safe? Safety may be one issue that some have, but we just took care of that one.

Pediatricians and medical doctors also may say it doesn't work. Again, let's use our logic. Starting from birth, think about all of the trauma and stress that your kids have put on their bodies. First the delivery, then learning to crawl and walk, all along the way falling all over the place. Do you think maybe their bodies and spines may get out of balance? Of course they can! They have nervous systems, too, right? So going back, if their spine gets out of place from all this stress and puts pressure on their nervous system, they aren't going to be as healthy. They can get symptoms like colic, constipation, reflux, ear infections, asthma like symptoms, and even headaches for the older kids. To be completely blunt, many pediatricians do things every day that have been proven not to work, like give antibiotics for ear infections. I bet you didn't know that. So bottom line, and this is not what we're shooting for, at worst, chiropractic care may not help them, but it definitely won't harm them. It's a natural, drug-free way to help their health, so why not give it a try, especially if nothing else has worked for your kids' health problems.

Q: What happens when my insurance runs out and won't pay for my care anymore? What if I can't afford it?

A: That's a very good question that we get a lot. It's called health insurance but it really isn't for health. They should call it sick insurance or pain insurance because that's what the insurance will pay

172

for. If treatment is to prevent disease or injuries, promote health, improve your overall health and well-being, the insurance <u>won't</u> pay for it. That's taken right from Medicare's guidelines. I'm not making it up. Once you hear it and read it, it sounds ridiculous, doesn't it? At least it does to me. Isn't that what you want – to prevent disease, promote health, and improve your overall well-being? Insurance definitely has its place and it's nice to have, but you can't count on it to get you healthy if that is your goal. If you truly want to get healthy, you might have to pay a little more out of your pocket for it.

The patients who can see down the road six months, a year, even two years, can see if they pay a little more out of their pocket now, get healthy, and maintain what they've accomplished, they are the ones that are the happiest and healthiest because they don't have headaches every day anymore, or they don't get sick as often, their allergies are better, or whatever it is. I think my own situation is similar to health and getting healthy, but mine has to do with yard work and landscaping. I do not like to do that stuff. I'll mow the lawn and weed whack and that's about it. My yard needs some work, but I look at it and I don't even know where to start. That's where I need some actual professional help. Have them fix it up nice and I'll maintain it with periodic help from the landscapers. I know I'll have to pay a little more, but at least I'll know it's going to get done right in a reasonable amount of time. It is the same thing with health. You might have to use some of your money to get healthy, but once you do, you'll be healthier and happier and have to pay less in the future to maintain it. We often overestimate what we can do in two months, but underestimate what we can accomplish in one, two, or three years. I know in our office, if you truly cannot afford it and you're committed to getting healthy, we will come up with a plan that you can afford. We don't want money to be the limiting factor in you getting healthy.

Q: Is it OK for me to see my medical doctor and see what he says? What if my medical doctor tells me not to see a chiropractor?

A: It's fine if you want to see your medical doctor. The only thing I have to say is that, in general, they don't treat muscle, nerve and bone problems every day, like we do. If you go in for low back pain or neck pain, more than likely he will prescribe some muscle relaxers or pain killers for the pain, but he will not get to the cause of the pain.

That leads to your next question, what if he tells you not to see a chiropractor. If it were me, I would ask why not. If he says he just doesn't like chiropractors or thinks we don't do anything, ask how he knows, or if he's ever been to a chiropractor or even talked to one before. If not, he's not a very reliable source. Just like if I told you to not go see your doctor if you had a flesh-eating bacteria because I just didn't like medical doctors. What would you think? You'd think I was crazy. Again, all of this information is IN GENERAL. There are many medical doctors who refer to chiropractors and vice versa, working tandem to improve their patient's health. Just like I can't say exactly what your medical doctor would do, it's difficult for them to know exactly what we do.

All day, chiropractors deal with muscle, bone, and nerve problems. Obviously, just through sheer practice and seeing these problems every day, we know what we're doing. So bottom line, you just need to use your common sense and judgment to come to the right conclusion. Believe me, I know it's hard to go against someone in an authoritative position when they say don't do something.

What about kids? We hear that a lot, too, with pediatricians not referring to chiropractors. Again, much of the problem exists because medical doctors don't know what we do, especially with kids. I don't know if they think we're going to rip their heads off or what, but we're not stupid. We use gentle techniques to help their bodies heal. If you're worried about injuring your babies or children, they might not have ever come out of the birth canal. Think about how traumatic that was with the doctor pulling on their head, pulling their shoulder down. We don't come anywhere near that type of force with treatment. But guess what? By being born, that proves that their bodies are strong and we can't do anything to hurt them using the techniques we use. If the problem is that they think chiropractors don't help with childhood problems, I can give a health report and various studies that show how chiropractic does help, especially for ear infections and colds. Some of the things medical doctors do are proven not to be effective, but they still do it. I really don't want to sling mud at anybody, but I also don't want to just stand there and get pelted with mud myself. I feel it's our duty to give you this information because you're not getting it anywhere else.

Q: *I know you're not a medical doctor, so how much education do you actually have?*

A: Actually, our education compares very well with medical doctors. Not many people know that, and sometimes we are even the butt of some jokes: "We are not 'real' doctors." But when you look at it, and the number of hours chiropractors and medical doctors spend on various subjects, chiropractors come out ahead in a lot of areas, especially in those areas that we treat and see every day like muscle, joint, and nerve problems.

Now I'm going to throw some numbers at you. A study done back in 1995 showed that chiropractic schools taught 875 hours of anatomy and physiology, compared to 510 hours in medical school. That's 365 more hours that chiropractors learned about muscles, joints, and nerves and how they work! And for the overall education curriculums, chiropractors had 155 more contact hours with various subjects and clinical experience. A survey of 18 chiropractic colleges and 22 medical schools was also done. Just to get their degrees, chiropractors needed 439 hours of orthopedic and x-ray, while medical students needed, are you ready, only 15 hours in those fields.

The last boring study I'll refer to was actually done by the *Journal of Bone and Joint Surgery*, a medical journal. Back in 1998, they tested recent medical school graduates in basic competency in musculoskeletal medicine. That's a long word for treating people with muscle and joint problems. They asked 124 orthopedic program directors to validate the study, which they did, and set the passing score at 73.1%. Well, 82% of the recent graduates failed to demonstrate basic competency in musculoskeletal medicine, not advanced knowledge, but basic competency. So they revisited this in 2002 thinking, well let's ask program directors for internal medicine departments and see if they can validate this test. So 240 internal medicine program directors looked at the test and gave an acceptable passing score of 70%. Using this percentage, 78% of the recent medical graduates still failed in basic competency. Remember, this is for musculoskeletal medicine. That's pretty amazing, and not many people know about these figures. I'm not trying to bash medicine, although I know it sounds like it. I

177

just want to give you the facts about chiropractic education to show you that we are on the same footing as medical doctors, or maybe even a little better equipped, especially when it comes to treating muscle, joint, and nerve problems.

Q: What can I do at home to help my spine and health?

A: You know, my hope is that everybody asks that question. When it comes down to it, it's what you do, not what we do. This is the compilation of what we've been talking about. To help with your health, you have to identify the physical, chemical, and emotional stresses that you are putting on your body and counteract those with physical, chemical, and emotional treatments, for lack of a better word, to get and stay healthy. If you keep doing what you've been doing, you'll always get what you've already got. So physically look at yourself and what you do – at work, at home, driving, sitting, standing, lifting, walking, and sleeping. Chemically, what are you eating and drinking and not eating and not drinking? Are you drinking too much caffeine, soda, coffee, not enough water, or not taking vitamins? Are you smoking or drinking a lot of alcohol? Emotionally, how are you feeling? How do you react to stressful and even minor situations? Is your home life, work life, or family life getting you frustrated or worried? All of these things play into how your body heals because they put stress on your body and nervous system.

One thing we haven't talked about yet is how important it is to have the proper curve in your neck. Looking at you from the side on x-ray, your neck, your spinal curve, should look like a C or the shape of a banana. If it's straight or going in the opposite direction, that puts pressure on the spinal cord. What causes the curve to go in the opposite direction? You guessed it – physical, chemical, and emotional stress. A neurosurgeon, Dr. Alfred Brieg, actually proved that when your neck is straight, it can stretch your spinal cord 5-7 cm, about 2-3 inches, and that change can cause disease. He didn't say pain, headaches, muscle tension. He said disease. So that could mean getting colds frequently, allergies, asthma, reflux, stomach problems, high blood pressure, or diabetes. And you know why that is now, right? To me, it makes sense how that can cause "diseases" like these. And I hope it makes sense to you now, too, because we keep talking about when the nervous system is not working properly, you can get symptoms, and the spinal cord is one of the main structures of the nervous system.

Something you can do at home in conjunction with your adjustments is use a traction device to correct the direction of your neck curve. What we use a lot in our office is called a neck orthotic, and all you do is lie on it, with it under your neck. We're counteracting two stresses with this one tool –

179

physical stress on your spine and emotional stress because you have to lie down and just relax while you do it. We already talked about a couple of other things you need to do, and that's exercise regularly and fix your poor eating habits. I don't like using the word diet, because in my mind that conjures up short-term images like the juice diet or the belly fat diet. I'm talking lifestyle changes for the long term. There are definitely things you can do on your own to help your health and take stress off your body.

Q: Why do I still have the pain or tightness right after I get adjusted?

A: Many times patients come in for treatment and they have tenderness in some muscles. We adjust them and the tenderness is still there. The pain and tenderness is still there because you have to give your body a chance, and time, to heal. Let's say you exercise for an hour, but you weighed yourself right after you worked out and you didn't lose any weight. Why not? Because you have to give your body a chance to adapt. Let's do another example, because I like examples. I use this one a lot. If I, or you, stuck a nail in your leg, it would hurt, right? If you took the nail out, would the pain go away immediately? Or let's say you hit your finger with a hammer. The hammer caused the pain, but it's not on your thumb anymore. So why should it still hurt? I think you know why. Those things caused <u>damage</u> to your body, so it's going to take time to heal. Just like when your spine and posture are less than desirable, they cause damage to your nervous system and muscles. The adjustment helps with the cause, your spine and posture alignment, but it takes time for the damages to your muscles, nerves, and ligaments to get better. Makes sense, doesn't it? That's why we say, and know, that just like it took time for your body to get out of alignment, it's going to take time to correct it.

TOTAL HEALTH RECOMMENDS...

Posture Supports

Powerstep® Foot Orthotics

A prescription-like arch support encased in a unique double-layer cushioned insole, plus a contoured stabilizing heel cup to balance your foundation. It provides effective relief for heel and arch pain, heel spurs, plantar fasciitis, neuromas, metatarsalgia, knee pain, hip pain, low back pain, and many other conditions.

*Foot Levelers Foot Orthotics (Spinal Pelvic Stabilizers)

Shoe inserts that support all three arches in your feet, thereby creating a stable foundation upon which to build proper body posture. Custom-made Foot Levelers are individualized to stabilize your spine and pelvis by correcting imbalances in your feet— the foundation of your skeletal system. Foot Levelers products offer therapy for low back pain, poor posture, hip and knee pain, neck pain, sacroiliac (SI) joint pain, and much more.

Cervical Pillow

Ergonomically designed to properly align your head and neck with your spine. Reduces pressure on the head and neck for a better night's rest and fewer aches and pains when rising out of bed in the morning. *Recommended if you sleep on your back.*

Water Pillow

Has the ability to provide continuous support of the neck. Water pillows provide relief from neck and back pain, headaches, snoring, muscle tension, temporomandibular joint (TMJ) syndrome, and sleeplessness. *Recommended if you sleep on your side or back.*

Lumbar Seated Support

Fills the gap between the lower spine and the seat back, helping to promote the natural lordosis (or curve), complement forward pelvic tilting, and inhibit slouching. Aids in providing relief, preventing future injury, and helping patients feel more comfortable.

Postural Correction

Foot Scan

Allows you to see the imbalances you have at the foundation of your body. These imbalances may occur even if you're not experiencing foot pain. Though they may go unnoticed, these imbalances contribute to postural misalignments, pain in areas throughout your body, and fatigue.

Corrective Postural Exercises

Exercises specific for your postural abnormalities to strengthen weak areas and stretch tight areas in order to balance and reshape your spine.

*Corrective Neck Support

The Posture Right™ by Neck Orthotic, Inc. helps correct the loss of cervical curve and forward head posture. Benefits problems such as neck pain, headaches, TMJ dysfunction, stress, breathing, and fatigue.

*Corrective Lumbar Support

Perfect for poor low back posture and low back pain. Helps to restore the low back lordosis, taking stress off the bones, ligaments, muscles, and nerves.

*Corrective Mid Back Arch

Used to care for slouched mid back and shoulders as well as forward head posture. Made of firm foam, they are ideal for stretching the spine and restoring curvature to your back and neck.

Exercise Tools

Foam Roll

Uses deep compression to roll out the muscle spasms that develop over time. This loosens the muscle, relaxes the nerves, increases blood flow, and aids in recovery.

Exercise/Stability Ball

Provides numerous benefits that range anywhere from rehabilitating back, hip, and knee injuries to delivering a powerful workout to improve core stability, posture, and muscle balance. You also improve your flexibility and your cardiovascular system by using a low-impact workout.

Medicine Ball

Medicine balls are a great multi-purpose training tool that can be used alone or with a partner to improve core strength, functional movements, reaction time, and coordination. Medicine ball training, in conjunction with a program of weight training and circuit training, can be used to develop strength and power.

Weighted Vest

Many athletes, firefighters, and other people whose physical stature is important to their performance, use weighted vests to train. Weighted vests are available in many different weight options. A 10-pound vest is standard, but 20-pound maximums are also available. Others can be found in much larger weights, for example, 40-pound maximums and even more.

Stretch/Resistance Bands

Resistance band exercises are ideal for home exercise programs and can easily be incorporated into a circuit-training format, helping to condition cardiovascular system and strengthen specific muscle groups. Because resistance tubing is so compact and lightweight, it can be used while away from home.

Pull Up Bar

I recommend the Door Gym or Iron Gym because they are designed to fit in most doorway frames or sit on the floor for pushups, dips, and sit-ups. Strengthen your back, biceps, and other upper body muscles without having to screw anything into the wall. When installed in the doorway, the device lets you perform pull-ups and chin-ups, with three grip positions -- narrow, neutral, and wide -- for working the inner and outer back. Once you're done with your back workout, you can move it to the floor, where you can perform pushups while facing down, triceps dips while facing the other way, or sit-ups using it for foot stability.

Palliative Care

Massage Therapy

Helps you relax, re-align and rejuvenate. There are many positive aspects to receiving massage therapy on an ongoing basis. With the busy lives we lead, we can all benefit from a little stress-management. Medical, deep tissue, sports, manual, lymphatic drainage, and prenatal are common types of massage.

Biofreeze

A greaseless, stainless, pain relieving gel with a vanishing scent. It provides temporary relief from minor aches and pains of sore muscles and joints associated with arthritis, backache, sprains and strains.

Ice Packs

Ice is one of the simplest, safest, and most effective self-care techniques for injury, pain, or discomfort in muscles and joints. Ice will decrease muscle spasms, pain, and inflammation to bone and soft tissue. You can use ice initially at the site of discomfort, pain, or injury. You can also apply ice in later stages for rehabilitation of injuries or chronic (long-term) problems.

Nutritional Support

Total Health Lifestyle Nutrition Manual

This book addresses the essential topic of incorporating healthy nutrition habits into your lifestyle. In it you'll find information on carbohydrates, protein, fat, shopping tips, easy food substitutions, and over 80 healthy recipes.

High Quality Multivitamin & Multimineral

A high quality multivitamin and multimineral is an excellent way to help restore your body's balance of vitamins and minerals and help you keep your normal pace.

Antioxidants

Antioxidants help neutralize free radicals, maximizing the body's ability to maintain health. This antioxidant activity supports energy levels and maintains optimal joint and cardiovascular health. Antioxidant supplementation goes beyond taking an ordinary multi-vitamin.

Omega-3 Fish Oil

Essential Omega-3 helps maintain healthy triglyceride and cholesterol levels by providing Omega-3 fatty acids and beneficial fish oils, which have been clinically demonstrated to provide a host of benefits that successfully promote cardiovascular health.

Probiotics

Today's diet consists of foods that may be designed and processed to extend shelf life. Though these foods are convenient, they can hinder the body's ability to efficiently digest and reap the nutritional compounds necessary for health. Probiotics replenish the essential enzymes and "good" bacteria necessary for maximum absorption of nutrients from the food we eat.

*Pro Enz

Pro-Enz is formulated for extended nutritional support of inflammation management. The combination of bromelain (plant-based proteolytic enzyme) and other key ingredients make it ideal for long-term maintenance. Pro-Enz is recommended for follow up after the acute phase of injury is addressed, as support for patients with physically demanding lifestyles (heavy labor, athletes) as well as those subject to pro-inflammatory lifestyle factors (poor diet, stress, etc.)

*Zymain

Designed to provide a nutritional foundation to the healing response following trauma, optimizing injury rehabilitation. Has been found to shorten rehabilitation time.

Vitamin C

Benefits include protection against immune system deficiencies, cardiovascular disease, prenatal health problems, eye disease, and even skin wrinkling.

B Complex

B vitamins play a vital role in maintaining body cell function. They are essential in every cell and tissue. Tissues in the nervous system, intestinal tract, and bone marrow tissues are the first to show signs of B-12 and folate deficiency. Vitamin B Complex provides optimal amounts of vitamin B12, B6, and folate, which contribute to numerous processes that help maintain proper cardiovascular and overall health.

Calcium

Your bones are the support structure holding up your body. Without calcium, bones and teeth can lose their health. Calcium supplements can give you an effective level of calcium to help you maintain healthy bones and teeth.

Nutritional Analysis

The Nutri-Physical is a free, internet-based analysis tool that recommends a customized nutritional supplementation program to improve an individual's quality of life.

* Denotes only to be used by prescription or under the supervision of a doctor.

www.TotalHealth-Fitness.com

Health & Fitness Programs

Many workout programs require you to progress from one
level to the next, and that is great! The problem is, many
times life gets in the way. These workouts are a little
different. Variety is important because it's boring doing the
same thing every time. Most of these programs don't require
you to progress from one level to the next. You pick which
one you want to do and you do it! Some are less intense than
others, and that's a good thing. Not all workouts should be
grueling.

Exercise Video Library

Gain access to a growing video library of exercises (over 115
different exercises and counting). It's broken up into different
sections so you can identify the exercises you want to learn
and perform. The sections are based on movement, not
muscle groups as is commonly seen.

Weekend Warrior Workouts

More than likely you have never been a professional athlete
and neither have we. We don't want to spend hours in the
gym, nor do we have the time. However, we want to improve
our performance in the sports that we like to play, just like
you.

Time Crunch Workout System

Everybody wants to be healthy. Too many do not want to do
the work. This workout program is specifically designed for

the busy person, especially parents, professionals, and travelers. Because we live in a busy world with tons of responsibilities, it is not practical for many of you to spend one to two hours every other day at the gym (commute time included). What you need is a logical, sensible workout program that makes it easy to workout.

Total Health Insider Newsletter

FREE Powerful Insider Tips to Achieve Your Optimal Health Potential.

Health and Wellness Articles

Learn about antibiotics, ADHD, drugs, asthma, cholesterol, common colds, flu shots, obesity, vaccines, osteoporosis, over-the-counter drugs, children's health, and almost every other health concern in this section.

The 38 Best Darn Ways to Avoid Sports Injuries eBook

Learn How to Prevent Your Nagging, Lingering, Sport Altering Injuries for FREE!

How to Build the Ultimate Young Athlete eBook

An Amazing Resource Focused 100% on Improving Athletic Ability for All Young Athletes!

SOURCES

Chapter 1: What is Health?
Lipton, Bruce H. *The Biology of Belief: Unleashing the Power of Consciousness, Matter, & Miracles*. India. Hay House. 2008.

Starfield, B. M.D. (2000, July 26). Is US health really the best in the world? *Journal of the American Medical Association,* July 26, 2000; 284(4), 483-485.

UCLA Center for Human Nutrition: http://www.cellinteractive.com/ucla/physcian_ed/stages_change.html.

WebMD: http://www.webmd.com/fitness-exercise/features/six-steps-that-can-change-your-life.

Chapter 2: Achieve Physical Balance and Alignment
Functional Movement Screen: www.FunctionalMovement.com.

Gutmann, G. The atlas fixation syndrome in the baby and infant. *Manuelle Medizin*. 1987; 25: 5-10.

Kendall FP, McCreary EK, Provance PG. *Muscles Testing and Function: Fourth Edition with Posture and Pain.* Williams & Wilkins. Baltimore, MD. 1993.

Towbin, A. "Latent Spinal Cord and Brain Stem Injury in Newborn Infants." *Developmental Medicine and Child Neurology.* 11:54-68. 1969.

Chapter 3: Exercise: Life is Movement
American Diabetes Association. http://www.diabetes.org/diabetes-statistics/cost-of-diabetes-in-us.jsp.

American Heart Association. *Heart Disease and Stroke Statistics — 2009 Update.* http://www.cdc.gov/NCCDPHP/publications/AAG/dhds p_text.htm#2.

Arthritis and Rheumatism 2007;56(5):1397–1407. http://www.cdc.gov/ARTHRITIS/data_statistics/faqs/cos t_analysis.htm.

Centers for Disease Control and Prevention. Budget Request Summary: Fiscal Year 2008. www.cdc.gov/fmo/PDFs/FY08_Budget_Summary_Final .pdf.

Centers for Disease Control and Prevention: http://www.cdc.gov/nccdphp/publications/factsheets/Prevention/obesity.htm.

Journal of Clinical Oncology, Vol 22, No 17 (September 1), 2004: pp. 3524-3530.

Psychology Today Magazine, Dec 2003
Last Reviewed 27 Jun 2005
http://www.psychologytoday.com/articles/pto-20040206-000005.html.

Stewart WF, PhD, MPH, et al. Lost Productive Time and Cost Due to Common Pain Conditions in the US Workforce. *Journal of the American Medical Association,* November 12, 2003;290:2443-2454.

Chapter 5: Mental Balance and Alignment: De-stress, not Distress
Carlson, Richard PhD. *Don't Sweat the Small Stuff...and it's all small stuff.* Hyperion. New York. 1997.

Davich, Victor. *8 Minute Meditation: Quiet Your Mind. Change Your Life.* Penguin Group. New York. 2004.

Dyer, Wayne. *The Power of Intention: Learning to Co-create Your World Your Way.* Hay House, Inc. California. 2004.

Chapter 6: Children's Health: What They Aren't Telling You

Cantekin, E.I. et. al. Antimicrobial therapy for otitis media with effusion ('secretory' otitis media). *Journal of American Medical Association.* Dec 1991. 266(23).

Coyle, J. (2000). Psychoactive drug use in very young children. Editorial. Journal of the American Medical Association, 283. Retrieved February 23, 2000 from http://jama.ama-assn.org/issues/v283n8/ffull/jed90109.html.

Damoiseaux RAMJ, van Balen FAM, Hoes AW, et al. Primary care based randomized, double blind trial of amoxicillin versus placebo for acute otitis media in children aged under 2 years. *British Medical Journal,* Feb. 5, 2000:320, pp350-54.

DiFiori, John, MD. Overuse Injuries in Children and Adolescents. *Phys Sportsmed* 1999; 27(1).

FDA Advisory warning: Antidepressant Use in Children, Adolescents and Adults: http://www.fda.gov/cder/drug/antidepressants/default.htm.

FDA. Antidepressant 'Black Box' label warning http://www.fda.gov/cder/drug/antidepressants/SSRIlabel Change.htm.

Freudenheim M. Behavior Drugs Lead in Sales for Children, New York Times, May 17, 2004. http://www.nytimes.com/2004/05/17/business/17drug.html?ex=1085815432&ei=1&en=72cd66cf54ffd8d4.

Garbutt JM, Goldstein M, Gellman E, et al. A randomized, placebo-controlled trial of antimicrobial treatment for children with clinically diagnosed acute sinusitis. *Pediatrics* 2001:107(4), pp. 619-625.

Grasso, B et al. *Development Essentials: The Foundations of Youth Conditioning.* International Youth Conditioning Association. 2005.

Grinfeld, M. 1998. Psychoactive medications and kids: New initiatives launched. Psychiatric Times. Vol 14 (3) March: p. 69.

Kraemer William, Fleck Steven. *Strength Training for Young Athletes.* Human Kinetics, Champaign, IL, 1993.

LeFever GB, Dawson KV, Morrow AL. The extent of drug therapy for attention deficit-hyperactivity disorder among children in public schools. *American Journal of Public Health*, Sept. 1999:89(9), pp1359-64.

Little et. al. "Pragmatic randomized controlled trial of two prescribing strategies for childhood acute otitis media." *British Medical Journal.* 2001; 322; 336-342.

Mangione-Smith R, McGlynn E, Elliott M, et al. The relationship between perceived parental expectations and pediatrician antimicrobial prescribing behavior. *Pediatrics*, April 1999:103(4), pp711-718.

Medco Health Solutions, Inc. 2004 Drug Trend Symposium. Study Reveals Pediatric Spending Spike on Drugs to Treat Behavioral Problems, May 17, 2004. http://biz.yahoo.com/prnews/040517/nym080_1.html.

Mendelsohn Robert MD. *How to Raise a Healthy Child in Spite of Your Doctor.* Ballantine Books. New York. 1984.

Strayhorn, CK. Forgotten children, Texas Comptroller, April 2004. http://www.window.state.tx.us/forgottenchildren/execsu mm/.

Towbin, A. "Latent Spinal Cord and Brain Stem Injury in Newborn Infants." *Developmental Medicine and Child Neurology.* 11:54-68. 1969.

Wagner KD, Ambrosini P, Rynn M, et al: Efficacy of sertraline in the treatment of children and adolescents with Major Depressive Disorder. JAMA 2003; 290(8):1033-1041.

Watson RL, Dowell SF, Jayaraman M, et al. Antimicrobial use for pediatric upper respiratory infections: reported practice, actual practice, and parent beliefs. *Pediatrics*, Dec. 1999:104(6), pp1251-57.

World Health Report, 1996. World Health Organization.

See also: Emslie GJ, Rush AJ, Weinberg WA, et al (1997b). A double-blind, randomized, placebo-controlled trial of fluoxetine in children and adolescents with depression. Arch Gen Psychiatry 54:1031-7; Keller, MB, Ryan ND, Stober M, et al.: Efficacy of paroxetine in the treatment of adolescent major depression: a randomized, controlled trial. J AM Acad Child Adolesc Psychiatry 2001; 40(7):762-772.

ABOUT THE AUTHOR

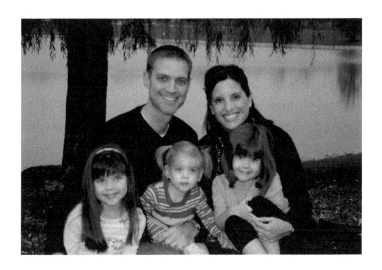

Dr. Ryan Wohlfert has been involved with health and fitness since he was a kid playing baseball, basketball, football, kick ball, whiffle ball, and everything else in his backyard. He wasn't doing it because he thought it was good for him. It was fun and he liked it. Unfortunately, that type of activity is giving way to sedentary activities in America: computer games, Internet surfing, TV watching, and texting. Over the last 17 years, his passion and purpose have evolved into helping as many people as possible learn about health and how to get healthy.

Dr. Ryan (as he is known to his patients) grew up in a small town that taught values, discipline, and hard work. He learned most of those attributes from his parents and community. His drive and ambition were formed at an early age, much of it due to his older brother. He wanted to perform at his absolute best, leading him to various accomplishments athletically and academically, including academic all-state and high school valedictorian.

His future ambitions were shaped during his senior year of high school. He realized he wanted to help people improve physically, so he studied Movement Science in the Division of Kinesiology at the University of Michigan, from which he graduated Summa Cum Laude with his first Bachelor's of Science degree. Because of Dr. Ryan's past experiences and desire to stay involved in athletics, he chose to become a chiropractor. He went to National College of Chiropractic (now National University of Health Sciences) in Lombard, Illinois, to continue his education, where he earned a second Bachelor's of Science degree and graduated Summa Cum Laude with his Doctorate of Chiropractic.

After graduation, he moved to Cary, North Carolina, where he and his wife ran a successful practice from 2000 through 2006. Although he and his family enjoyed their time there, they were 800 miles away from their family and decided to move back to Michigan in late 2006.

In addition to being a Doctor of Chiropractic, Dr. Ryan also earned his Certifications as a Strength and Conditioning Specialist and a Chiropractic Sports Physician, and is in Advanced Standing as a Youth Conditioning Specialist. He works with local high school athletes to improve their performance, prevent injuries, and instill a lifelong habit of healthy activities.

Today, Dr. Ryan and his wife, Dr. Monica, own Total Health Chiropractic, a community leader in health care and education in Lansing and Westphalia. Their passion is to help families and their community become physically, chemically, and mentally balanced (i.e. Get Healthy) through chiropractic care, exercise instruction, nutritional counseling, and de-stressing techniques. Their goal is to make a positive difference in the lives they touch.

Dr. Ryan and Dr. Monica have 3 little girls, Rylee, Dylan, and Kaelyn. With their work in their practice and community, they hope to leave a legacy for their family that will last for generations.

"What we have done for ourselves alone dies with us. What we have done for others lasts forever."

CPSIA information can be obtained
at www.ICGtesting.com
Printed in the USA
LVHW011434190821
695682LV00020B/838